DR. MORRISON'S HEART-SAVER PROGRAM

DR. MORRISON'S
HEART-SAVER PROGRAM

A NATURAL, SCIENTIFICALLY TESTED PLAN FOR THE PREVENTION OF ARTERIOSCLEROSIS, HEART ATTACK, AND STROKE

by Lester Morrison, M.D., D.Sc., F.A.C.P.
Director of the Institute for Arteriosclerosis Research

WITH NANCY NUGENT

ST. MARTIN'S PRESS ● NEW YORK

Library of Congress Cataloging in Publication Data

Morrison, Lester M.
    Dr. Morrison's Heart-saver program.

    Bibligraphy: p.
    Includes index.
    1. Arteriosclerosis—Prevention.   2. Heart—Diseases—
Prevention.   3. Aging—Prevention.   I. Nugent, Nancy.
II. Title.   III. Title: Heart-saver program.
RC692.M65   1983   616.1'05   82-11301
ISBN 0-312-21481-2

First Edition
10 9 8 7 6 5 4 3 2 1

This research, book and health program are dedicated to my wife, Rita, and to the memories of my parents and my wife's parents—each of whom died from the ravages of arteriosclerosis and its complications (heart attack, stroke).

A Note to the Reader

TABLE OF CONTENTS

ACKNOWLEDGMENTS

To Mary Cannon, B.A., for her secretarial assistance; Monica Stevens, B.A., and Janet Brown, B.A., for their years of laboratory and technical assistance; Irene Parks, for her many years of dietary, menu and recipe assistance on the low-fat, low-cholesterol diet; William Gottlieb, our editor at Rodale Press, for his indefatigable and creative suggestions regarding the manuscript; Christy Kohler of Rodale Press for her research assistance; Norbert H. Enrick, Ph.D., our invaluable statistical colleague; and many others so numerous that space limitations prevent our mentioning them. The following list credits fifty-six scientific coinvestigators and colleagues whose work has provided the foundation for the research findings and programs of the Institute for Arteriosclerosis Research. In addition to the scientists and physicians on this rather extensive list, there are a number of other practicing physicians who have contributed to our research program—either as patients themselves or as collaborators—to whom we are grateful.

INVESTIGATORS AND CONSULTANTS

Institute for Arteriosclerosis Research
Loma Linda University School of Medicine
University of California
University of Southern California

PAST AND CURRENT

L. M. Morrison, M.D. Principal Investigator, President, Director and Research Professor, Institute for Arteriosclerosis Research, Loma Linda University School of Medicine, Loma Linda, California; Consultant in Medicine, University of California Center for Health Sciences, Los Angeles.

B. H. Ershoff, Ph.D. Scientific Director, Institute for Arteriosclerosis Research; Research Professor of Biochemistry, Loma Linda University School of Medicine, Loma Linda, California; Emeritus Professor, University of Southern California School of Medicine, Los Angeles.

K. Murata, M.D., Ph.D. Assistant Professor of Medicine, University of Tokyo School of Medicine, Tokyo, Japan; Visiting Assistant Professor of Medicine and Research Associate, Institute for Arteriosclerosis Research, Loma Linda University School of Medicine, Loma Linda, California.

J. J. Quilligan, Jr., M.D. Professor of Pediatrics Research, Virus and Infectious Diseases, Loma Linda University School of Medicine, Loma Linda, California; Life Career Investigator, NIH.

O. A. Schjeide, Ph.D. Chief and Associate Professor, Metabolic Section, Radiobiology Division, Laboratory of Nuclear Medicine and Radiation Biology, University of California Center for Health Sciences, Los Angeles. xiii

N. H. Enrick, Ph.D.   Professor of Statistics, Business
Management School, Kent State University, Kent, Ohio.

G. S. Bajwa, D.V.M., Ph.D.   Research Associate, Institute
for Arteriosclerosis Research, Los Angeles; formerly
Instructor and Veterinarian, Department of Veterinary
Bacteriology, Washington State University, Pullman, and
Michigan State University, East Lansing.

R. B. Alfin-Slater, Ph.D.   Professor of Nutrition and Public
Health Nutrition, University of California Center for
Health Sciences, Los Angeles.

J. C. Roberts, M.D.   Assistant Clinical Professor of
Pathology, University of California Center for Health
Sciences, Los Angeles; Director of Research, Little
Company of Mary Hospital, Torrance, California.

S. Bernick, Ph.D.   Research Professor of Anatomy,
University of Southern California School of Medicine,
Los Angeles.

P. R. Patek, Ph.D.   Chairman and Professor, Department of
Anatomy, University of Southern California School of
Medicine, Los Angeles.

O. J. Dunn, Ph.D.   Professor of Biostatistics and
Biomathematics, Assistant Dean of Academic Affairs,
School of Public Health, Vice Chairman, School of Public
Health, University of California, Los Angeles.

M. R. Malinow, M.D.   Chairman, Division of Cardiovascular
Physiology, Oregon Regional Primate Research Center;
Associate Professor of Medicine, University of Oregon
School of Medicine, Portland.

H. Selye, M.D., Ph.D., D.Sc.   Professor and Director,
Institut de Medicine et de Chirurgie Experimentales,
University of Montreal, Montreal, Canada.

A. W. Branwood, M.D.   Acting Chairman and Associate
Professor of Pathology, New York Hospital, Cornell
Medical Center, New York City.

R. C. Robbins, Ph.D.   Associate Professor, Department of
Food Science, Institute of Food and Agricultural
Sciences, University of Florida, Gainesville.

L. O. Pilgeram, Ph.D. Director, Gerontology Research Institute, The Sansum Clinic Research Foundation, Santa Barbara, California; recently Professor and Director, Division of Arteriosclerosis Research, University of Minnesota, Minneapolis.

S. Renaud, Ph.D. Director, Laboratory of Experimental Pathology, Institut de Cardiologie de Montreal, University of Montreal, Montreal, Canada.

J. F. Prudden, M.D. Associate Professor of Surgery, Columbia University College of Physicians and Surgeons, New York City.

G. B. Jerzy Glass, M.D. Professor of Medicine, New York College of Medicine, New York City.

R. J. Veenstra, D.V.M. Director of Veterinary Services, Woodard Asiatic Corporation, San Francisco.

P. R. Rucker, M.S. Biochemist, Institute for Arteriosclerosis Research, Los Angeles.

A. T. Daugaard, M.S. Research Assistant in Histology, Institute for Arteriosclerosis Research, Los Angeles.

S. Srinivasan, Ph.D. Career Investigator, NIH, for New York City, Laboratory of Vascular Surgery, Department of Surgery, State University of New York, Downstate Medical Center, Brooklyn.

C. Simpson, D.V.M., Ph.D. Professor of Veterinary Medicine and Pathology, Department of Veterinary Science, University of Florida, Gainesville.

R. Hammer, Ph.D. Assistant Professor of Pharmacology and Molecular Biology, Department of Veterinary Science, University of Florida, Gainesville.

T. Pamer, Ph.D. Gastroenterology Research Division, Department of Medicine, New York College of Medicine, New York City.

M. Horowitz, M.D. Gastroenterology Research Division, Department of Medicine, New York College of Medicine, New York City.

D. Kritchevsky, Ph.D. Professor of Biochemistry, Wistar Institute of Anatomy and Biology, University of Pennsylvania, Philadelphia.

W. A. Loeven, Ph.D.   Career Investigator, NIH,
Gerontology Research Center, Baltimore City Hospitals,
Baltimore.

A. J. Seaman, M.D.   Research Professor of Hematology and
Medicine, University of Oregon, Portland.

W. Regelson, M.D.   Professor and Chairman, Department of
Medicine, Division of Medical Oncology, Medical College
of Virginia, Richmond.

K. Meyer, M.D., Ph.D.   Professor of Biochemistry, Columbia
University and Belfer Graduate School of Science,
Yeshiva University, New York City.

C. V. R. Born, Ph.D.   Professor and Director,
Pharmacological Institute, Royal College of Surgeons of
England, London.

S. Bazin, Ph.D.   Biochemist, Institut Pasteur, Garches, Haut-
de-Seine, France.

B. S. Bull, M.D.   Assistant Professor of Pathology, School of
Medicine, Loma Linda University, Loma Linda,
California.

M. H. Samitz, M.D.   Professor and Director, Division of
Graduate Medicine, Graduate Dermatology, University of
Pennsylvania School of Medicine, Philadelphia.

J. Green, Ph.D.   Head, Atherosclerosis Project, Beecham
Research Laboratores, Vitamin Research Station, Surrey,
England.

J. L. Gordon, Ph.D.   Department of Pathology, University of
Cambridge, Cambridge, England.

L. Robert, Ph.D.   Director, Laboratoire de Biochimie du
Tissu Conjonctif, Equipe de Recherche du CNRS, Paris.

H. C. Bergman, Ph.D.   Pharmacologist, Institute for
Arteriosclerosis Research, Los Angeles, California.

S. Gero, M.D.   Professor of Medicine and Chairman, Third
Department of Medicine, Semmelweis University,
Budapest, Hungary.

A. Bertelli, Ph.D.   Direttore, Universita' Degli Studi di Pisa,
Instituto di Farmacologia, Pisa, Italy.

I. F. Capdevielle, M.D. Hospital Municipal Guillermo Rawson, Departamente de Medicina, Unidad de Internacion No. 4 (Clinica B), University of Buenos Aires, Buenos Aires, Argentina.

M. Aylward, M.D. Director, Simbec Research Institute, Cefn Coed, Wales, U.K.

M. Cloarec, M.D. Professor, Hopital Saint-Antoine, Paris.

J. D. Romm, M.D. Assistant Professor of Medicine, University of California, Los Angeles.

J. K. Vyden, M.D. Associate Professor of Medicine, University of California, Los Angeles.

H. Rose, Ph.D. Assistant Director, Cardiovascular Rehabilitation Department, Cedars-Sinai Medical Center, Los Angeles.

A. N. Klimov, M.D., Ph.D. Director of Atherosclerosis Research, Institute for Experimental Medicine, Leningrad, USSR.

V. E. Ryzhenkov, M.D. Assistant Director, Laboratory of Experimental Therapy of Atherosclerosis, Institute for Experimental Medicine, Leningrad, USSR.

K. Schwarz, M.D., Ph.D. (deceased). Associate Professor of Biochemistry, University of California, Los Angeles; Chief, Laboratory of Experimental Metabolic Diseases, Veterans Administration Hospital, Long Beach, California.

B. Abuin de Leon, M.D. Research Department, Servicio de Neurologia, Hospital Espanol, Buenos Aires, Argentina.

S. Muchnik, M.D. Chief, Servicio de Neurologia, Hospital Espanol, Buenos Aires, Argentina.

Chapter 1

HEART ATTACK—IT CAN BE STOPPED BEFORE IT GETS STARTED

It's heartbreaking to see so many hearts breaking down—especially when I know this tragedy can be prevented.

I am Lester Morrison, M.D., and I have been a doctor for over fifty years. Much of that time has been devoted to finding a way to stop heart disease, which killed my mother, my father and several other members of my family and remains the number one killer in the United States and other developed countries. Now I'm writing to share with you the result of all that work, a result that I hope will help you and your loved ones to reduce the heart disease statistics by staying out of them. It's a preventive lifestyle called the Institute Program.

What Institute? I'm referring to the Institute for Arteriosclerosis Research whose research has been affiliated with the University of California of Los Angeles (UCLA), the University of Southern California, the Loma Linda University and numerous other universities and medical centers in this country and abroad. The Institute was founded as a nonprofit, charitable, medical research foundation by my wife, Rita, and me right after World War II for the purpose of studying, preventing and, we hope, treating and "curing" heart disease and other complications of arteriosclerosis (also known as atherosclerosis or hardening of the arteries).

Heart attacks don't just happen. They don't strike just anyone. They aren't contagious, and they aren't accidents. They are the result of a very specific series of events that occur throughout a person's life and can usually be counted on to build up to a heart attack in middle or old age—or perhaps even sooner. By preventing that series of events in your own life, you stand a good chance of preventing a heart attack.

Realistically, I cannot guarantee you that you'll never have a heart attack, even if you follow every bit of advice in this book. But I can promise you that if you read this book, understand it, and follow the carefully developed Institute Program, you can *lessen* your chances of having a heart attack (and even a stroke) and *increase* your chances of living a longer and healthier life.

You Are an Individual

Why can't I guarantee you that you won't have a heart attack? Because I don't know you. No responsible doctor would try to predict the health of a person he hasn't personally examined. There are just too many variables.

How old are you? Are you a man or a woman? Did your parents, grandparents, or great-grandparents have heart attacks? Where were you born? What kinds of food were you fed as a child? What do you eat now? What kind of work do you do? Are you under a great deal of constant emotional stress? Do you smoke a lot, a little, or not at all? Do you drink a lot of alcohol and coffee, a little, or none at all? Are you overweight, underweight, or just right? Is your blood pressure high, low, or normal? Do you exercise regularly? What diseases have you had up to now?

If you were my patient, I would ask you all these questions because many years of research have proved that the answers have a great deal to do with whether or not you, as an individual, will have a heart attack or stroke. Your answers would give me a pretty good idea of whether or not you were in a high-risk group. A physical examination would tell me much more. And the results of laboratory tests done on a sample of your blood would, with those other facts, tell me whether you were pretty safe from having a heart attack, about average, or in danger.

However, even if you were in the pretty safe group, I would still recommend that you follow the Institute Program.

Why? Because it's never too early and rarely too late to start a program of prevention.

Degenerative Diseases

Heart attacks don't happen overnight. They are not bolts out of the blue, and they are not an inescapable part of middle or old age. They are the result of a long and complicated series of degenerative diseases. These diseases begin in your childhood or youth; they work against your body for years and years; finally, they cause your heart to break down. Now we know that they can be prevented. They can be stopped before they get started. And here's even better news for adults: Even if they have already gotten started, in many cases they can be stopped before they have gone too far. And that's doubly important when you realize that most people who have these diseases don't have any idea how "far-gone" they are!

Most of us know or have heard of someone who's had a "sudden" heart attack. "I can't believe it!" his friends and family say in shock. "He was so healthy! Just yesterday he was perfectly all right, and today he dropped dead of a heart attack!"

Not quite. The truth is that such people were not "so healthy" or "perfectly all right." They just appeared to be well; the degenerative diseases that lead to arteriosclerosis, heart attack and stroke are so slow in development, so painless, and so free of symptoms that most people don't know they are under attack. But they are—slowly and quietly the diseases are marshaling their forces and lying in wait until . . . heart attack!

My work, and the work of countless other research scientists, has been devoted to one goal: discovering these degenerative diseases, learning everything there is to learn about them, and finding ways to stop them. When I say "countless," I'm quite serious. No one knows exactly how many scientists and physicians have given their time and energy to this fight, but we have all helped each other, as you'll see.

When one doctor or group of doctors makes a discovery, an account of it is published in one of many medical journals that scientists or physicians read. Most of these discoveries concern very small but important health factors and don't get reported in the media; you haven't heard of most of the magazines I'll mention. But the discoveries are important because they represent milestones along the way to greater medical knowledge. They are documented proof of work that has been done, ideas that have been tested and results that have been achieved.

The Institute Formula

I'm going to tell you about many of these documented proofs because I want you to understand that the Institute Program is not just a passing fad that has been dreamed up to capitalize on the current high level of interest in health. This is even more important with respect to the high point of the Institute Program—the Institute Formula.

The Institute Formula is the result of years of research by my associates and myself. The Institute Formula is not a drug; it is not a chemical. It is a natural food supplement. Everything in it comes from nature, and these ingredients have been extracted and blended together. The Institute Formula has been tested and retested, and numerous studies have been published in medical journals and textbooks to show that each of its ingredients is an effective preventive agent against the degenerative diseases that lead to arteriosclerosis, heart attack and stroke.

In this book I'm going to tell you everything there is to know about the Institute Formula, taking you step by step through the research and testing processes, showing you the proof of its effectiveness. I'm going to tell you not only *how* it works, but *why* it works—and how my coinvestigators and I discovered these facts. I'm also going to tell you about the other parts of the Institute Program, ways in which you can give yourself a good fighting chance against the tragedy of heart disease.

What You Can Expect

Here's what you'll find in this book:

In chapter 2, I will tell you about arteriosclerosis, a disease that is better known as "hardening of the arteries." It is extremely important because it is a heart attack's calling card. You'll learn what it is, how it begins, how it works, and what you can do to prevent it if you don't have it, or to stop it if you do.

Chapter 3 explains how I know that degenerative diseases can be prevented, and how our Institute and I discovered this fact. I'll tell you about some of my own research and the research of other scientists and doctors in the same field. I think it's very important that you know just how the Institute Program came about—and I think you'll find it interesting, too.

Chapters 4 and 5, the "heart" of the book, will analyze the Institute Formula, ingredient by ingredient, and tell you exactly how and why each of these ingredients is effective against degenerative diseases. You'll learn more about my work, some of my patients, my successes and failures, and the work of many other research scientists. When you've finished, you'll know everything there is to know about the Institute Formula.

Here comes another diet—haven't you had enough of them? Practically every health book you see these days tells you what you should and shouldn't eat, and this one is no different. But by the time you get to chapter 6 you'll know *why* diet is so important, and why your choice of foods may either help save your life—or help to kill you.

Then I'll tell you to get up from the table and stay up, at least long enough to give your body some exercise. Exercise may be boring—let's get that out of the way right at the start. But it's also necessary. I'll tell you why in chapter 7, and also give you some ideas for getting the amount you need *without* getting bored.

Chapter 8 will give you some up-to-date information on three very popular subjects of controversy—alcohol, caffeine and tobacco. Are they really as bad as most people say they are? Not necessarily. Do you have to give them up in order to prevent a heart attack? No. Alcohol and caffeine can even do you some good, although I don't hold out much hope for tobacco and certainly won't tell you to start smoking if you don't now. If you're already a smoker, though, you may not have to quit entirely. Chapter 8 will tell you why and help you to handle all three of these risky but well-loved habits.

Chapter 9 puts it all together—the Institue Program, how to use it, and what it can do for you. Based on our research, our statisticians give you an estimate of how many years you can add to your life when you follow the Institute Program. This can be up to 13.5 years!

How to Use This Book

When you were a child, your parents and teachers probably told you never to write in a book. I'm going to tell you just the opposite. I think you'll get a lot more out of this book if you go through it with a pen or pencil in hand. Underline words and sentences. Make notes in the margins. Write question marks if you don't understand something; when you find the answer, go back and write the answer's page number under the question mark.

Personalize this book by writing in facts about yourself that will make the general statements more meaningful to you as an individual. This is *your* book about *your* life—and it's *your* heart attack or stroke we're trying to prevent.

Good luck! I hope no heart specialist will ever have to treat you, no emergency room ever see you, no paramedic ever call you a "coronary" or "stroke." I hope you'll be able to live well into the twenty-first century, actively enjoying all the wonders that wait for us there. I hope you will be a slim, energetic, and healthful grandparent and great-grandparent, living to be part of an era in which heart disease will no longer be our nation's number one killer. And I hope, most of all, that this book can help you in achieving these goals.

Chapter 2

WHAT IS ARTERIOSCLEROSIS— AND WHY IS IT KILLING YOU?

Imagine driving through a tunnel at rush hour. Cars are lined up bumper to bumper, progress is slower than you'd like, but you are moving steadily forward. You'd better be, because you have an urgent appointment at the other end.

Suddenly a car some distance ahead of you stalls and comes to a stop. Its driver tries and tries, but can't get it started, and nothing can be done but wait for a tow truck. Tempers flare, people swear, and all the drivers behind the disabled vehicle start trying to edge their cars into the other lane to get around the blockage. The formerly smooth flow of traffic has become a snail's pace snarl, and everyone, no matter how much he wants to hurry, is going to have a slow, difficult time getting through the tunnel. It's enough to make you frantic, but there's nothing you can do about it.

The traffic jam is a lot like arteriosclerosis—but there *is* something you can do about that. Arteriosclerosis is the major cause of death in America today, but I'm going to tell you how to help keep yourself from being one of its victims.

How is arteriosclerosis like a traffic jam? The tunnel represents your arteries; the traffic is the blood that has to get through the arteries to keep your body alive. The stalled car   7 represents a collection of fatty material called an atherosclerotic plaque, and the result of this blockage is the same in both the tunnel and the arteries: flow is slowed down. The consequences, however, are far more serious in arteriosclerosis; although the slowing of traffic through a tunnel may cause anger, lateness, or a missed appointment, the slowing of blood through your arteries can—and often does—lead to death.

Just what is arteriosclerosis? Doctors sometimes call it "coronary artery disease" because it is usually found in the arteries that branch off from the heart. Most nonmedical people call it "hardening of the arteries," but that's only part of the problem. It should be called "clogging and hardening of the arteries," because the arteries don't get hard until globs of fat and scar tissue clog up their insides. Webster's Dictionary comes closer to the truth, defining arteriosclerosis as "a chronic disease characterized by abnormal thickening and hardening of the arterial walls." It's the abnormal thickening that impairs the blood flow and turns healthy, energetic people into sick, weak and eventually dead ones.

The word "arteriosclerosis" breaks down into two parts: "arterio" means "arteries," and "sclerosis" means "hardening." But why does it matter whether the arteries harden? Pipes are hard, but water still flows through them, and that traffic I mentioned would have a hard time making it through a soft-walled tunnel. However, when fatty material clogs the insides of arteries, which are really just very long tubes, the tubes also get narrower. Imagine trying to sip a drink through a regular straw, then switching to one of those little plastic swizzle sticks you get in mixed drinks in a bar. The smaller the tube, the bigger the difference—and the harder it is for the liquid to get through.

A glob of fatty material here and there won't make much difference. But a lot of globs, collected over a long time, create a thick inner lining, and blood can't get through the arteries as fast as the body needs it.

When the arteries are clogged and the flow of blood is slowed down, the body's organs can't get the oxygen they need, any more than a car's engine can get the gas it needs if the fuel line is clogged. The most important organ, of course, is the heart. Without oxygen and nutrients, the heart can't function. If the slowdown of blood flow gets serious enough, the heart has an "attack"—and everyone knows the results of a heart attack. You may survive one or even two; but eventually the heart can't take any more abuse and just gives out and stops.

So arteriosclerosis is hardening and narrowing of the arteries, with a slowdown of blood flow and a shortage of oxygen. It is the first step in the development of a heart attack.

Why Is Arteriosclerosis Killing You?

The question assumes that arteriosclerosis *is* killing you, which is a pretty serious statement. Unfortunately, there's a very good chance that it is true if you're an adult American. The chance is even greater if you're an American male, and greatest of all if you're an American male more than 40 years old.

Why American? Because our diets in this country contain more fat than most. The American diet is the second fattiest in the world; only Finland eats more fat then we do. Is it any wonder that the American death rate from arteriosclerosis and heart attacks is also in second place? In countries with especially low-fat diets—Greece, Yugoslavia and Japan, for instance—the death rates from these causes are 75 percent lower!

Why male? Because, in general, men's diets contain a lot more fat than women's do. Also, female hormones are thought to protect young women against arteriosclerosis. After the menopause, when natural production of these hormones slows down and stops, the protection also stops—but by that time a woman has had the benefit of it for about fifty years. Men die of heart attacks far more often than women do.

Why more than 40? Because it takes many fat globs to narrow an artery, and many years for the globs to collect and build up. The process begins at birth; by the time it becomes serious enough to cause a heart attack, the victim is usually more than 40 years old.

Chances are that arteriosclerosis is working on you right now and has been all your life. That's the bad news. The good news is that you may be able to stop it—you may even be able to reverse it—with the help of the Institute Formula. If you use the Formula according to my plan, and at the same time follow my low-fat diet and change your lifestyle for the better, you can improve the way you look and feel now and in the future. And that future may last a lot longer than it will if you let the fat keep building up in your arteries.

Arteriosclerosis is killing you because you have made the job so easy. It may be stopped if you take the steps to *make* it stop.

What Causes Arteriosclerosis?

It's easy to understand what arteriosclerosis *is*. But the way it gets started and grows is no simple matter. Your body is a very complicated machine, far more complicated than the engine of the car that caused the tunnel's traffic jam. Still, even with no medical background, you can understand how it develops and what brings it about. And once you understand how the enemy operates, the plan for defeating it will be a lot easier to follow.

The Most Dangerous Type

If you've ever heard a doctor mention the word "atherosclerosis," you've probably wondered whether it's the same thing as arteriosclerosis, and if it's not, what the difference is. Atherosclerosis is one type of arteriosclerosis, just as a sedan is one type of car. But atherosclerosis is the most common type of arteriosclerosis and also the most dangerous. It is the type that results from too much fat, the kind of fat that doctors call "lipids."

You can't live without lipids—they help to build cells all through your body—but you can't live with too much of them, either. You also have to know what kind of lipid you're dealing with; there are fatty lipids called cholesterol and triglyceride, and "detergent" lipids called *phospho*lipids.

Phospholipids. These substances are called "the blood's detergents" because they neutralize the fatty lipids and clean them out of your blood. Some of them are manufactured right in your body, by the liver. But you have to have enough of them to combat the amount of cholesterol you get from the foods you eat; you need a balance that changes every time you have a meal. This balance is called the "phospholipid:cholesterol ratio."

Luckily, phospholipids are also available in certain foods. If your liver is not producing enough to maintain a favorable phospholipid:cholesterol ratio, you can tip the balance in your favor by eating such foods as soybeans, whole wheat grains, certain nuts and other legumes. On the other hand, you can do exactly the opposite, and overload your body with cholesterol by eating egg yolks, butter, whole milk, cream and fatty meats. Sadly, this is what most Americans do.

A phospholipid called lecithin (described in chapter 4) is one of the most effective weapons against arteriosclerosis because it works directly against the condition called hyperlipidemia—very high levels of certain types of blood fats.

Cholesterol. This waxy substance is a solid fat that was first discovered in the examination of gallstones. Cholesterol moves through your bloodstream and is notorious for clinging to the walls of arteries, where it serves no useful purpose but builds up gradually over the years to create a fatty lining that hardens and narrows the inside walls.

You swallow great amounts of cholesterol every time you eat food that comes from animals: The heaviest sources of it are egg yolks, shrimp, whole milk products (butter, cheese, cream, ice cream) and red meats marbled with fat. Chances are these are some of your favorite foods. But you don't have to give them up—and you shouldn't—because cholesterol isn't all bad.

Triglyceride. This fatty lipid is the most common fat in food; it is present in vegetables as well as in animal products. But the difference between vegetable lipids and animal lipids is also the difference between two terms that have become household words in recent years: saturated and polyunsaturated fats.

What do "saturated" and "polyunsaturated" really mean? You hear them all the time, especially in TV commercials. The housewife says, "I cook with So-and-So's vegetable oil because it's polyunsaturated and helps my family in our fight against cholesterol." But did you notice that she says "oil" instead of "fat"? In those two words lies the difference between saturated and polyunsaturated.

Animal lipids are solid at room temperature and are called "fats." Almost all vegetable lipids are liquid at room temperature and are called "oils." The solid fats are saturated; they contain great amounts of cholesterol. The liquid oils are polyunsaturated and contain little or no cholesterol. In most cases, therefore:

Solid = Saturated = Cholesterol = Danger
Liquid = Polyunsaturated = No Cholesterol = Safety

Of course, a rule wouldn't be a rule without a few exceptions. Food scientists have found ways to make some solid fats with liquid vegetable oils, so we have polyunsaturated margarine and vegetable shortening. But to be safe, you have to read labels. Whenever you buy a solid fat, look for the key word "polyunsaturated" on the label. Then check the ingredient listing to be sure it says "cholesterol, 0 mg (milligrams)." If it does, buy it, use it and enjoy the knowledge that you're doing your arteries a favor.

Advertisers who claim that "saturated" is bad and "polyunsaturated" is good aren't making false statements. It's true they're trying to sell their products, but when they tell you to reduce your dietary intake of saturated fats, they should be believed and trusted.

On the other hand, don't think that complete elimination of lipids from your diet would be a good thing. The solution to the problem of fat buildup is not that simple. Some kinds of lipids carry energy that your body needs; lipids also help you to absorb vitamins A, D and E.

The key word is "moderation." Lipids are essential to life and health, but overdoing their use means undoing their benefits.

How Does the Body Use Lipids?

Generally, most fats can't move through the bloodstream on their own, any more than you could fly across the country on your own; they need protein to transport them just as you need an airplane. When you get on a plane you become an airplane passenger; a lipid that "gets on" a protein becomes a lipoprotein. This happens as you digest your food.

All lipoproteins contain triglyceride, cholesterol and phospholipid; but there are different amounts in the four different types of lipoprotein.

The four types are:

1. Chylomicrons
2. Very-low-density lipoproteins (VLDL)
3. Low-density lipoproteins (LDL)
4. High-density lipoproteins (HDL)

Chylomicrons. These are the largest lipoproteins. They are about 80 to 95 percent triglyceride, with very small amounts of cholesterol, phospholipid and protein.

Chylomicrons are the "airplane" that carries triglyceride from the food you eat out of your intestine and into your bloodstream. Its destination is the liver, where the triglyceride is converted into energy and used to build cells and provide body heat. Leftover chylomicrons are stored in the cells for later use in energy production. But everyone knows what happens if you keep stocking the coal bin without using the furnace.

VLDL. These lipoproteins are also mostly triglyceride (60 to 80 percent), but rather than coming from food, this form is usually manufactured by the liver. The VLDL carries this "homemade" triglyceride to fatty tissues, where it is used as energy or is stored. But in this case the leftovers don't build up; they go back to the liver, which uses them to make still more triglyceride. This is one of nature's recycling plans, and it's been around since long before humans thought of pulverizing old newspapers and pop-top cans.

LDL. This is the dangerous lipoprotein, the villain responsible for 50 to 60 percent of the blood's total cholesterol content, and for most of the cholesterol found in narrowed arteries. The LDL is mostly cholesterol and about 25 percent protein.

The LDL has a special transportation problem: It can get into an artery, but then it can't get out—somewhat like a finger carelessly stuck into the narrow neck of a bottle. Once it is trapped in the artery, the LDL "gives up" and disintegrates, and its cholesterol sticks to the walls of the artery, beginning or adding to a deadly buildup of fat.

HDL. This lipoprotein is mostly protein and phospholipid, with a small to moderate amount of LDL-cholesterol and very little triglyceride. Its claim to special attention is that *it is the only one of the four lipoproteins that is not usually linked to hyperlipidemia.*

Quite the contrary. There is strong evidence that HDL plays an important role in the removal of harmful lipids (like LDL) from the blood and the walls of the arteries, maybe because it contains phospholipid with "detergent" action. The HDL's are the good, protective forces.

Still, the prevention of hyperlipidemia is a matter of *balance.* The objective is to *increase* the level of protective HDL, *reduce* the amount of destructive LDL, and *utilize* the energy-producing qualities of the lipids you get from food.

Easy to say, but not so easy to do. Many years and the efforts of hundreds of research workers have been devoted to achieving this goal. That's what makes the Institute Formula so exciting: At long last, all this work has produced a *practical, readily available* and *effective* weapon against the chain reaction that starts with hyperlipidemia and progresses through arteriosclerosis to heart attack and death.

Who Gets Hyperlipidemia?

Usually, hyperlipidemia runs in families. That is, some people (really very few) inherit a tendency to collect excessive amounts of cholesterol and triglyceride in their bloodstreams. This type is called "primary" hyperlipidemia.

Other people retain fats as the result of diseases such as diabetes, gout and disorders of the gallbladder. In these cases, the hyperlipidemia is "secondary" to the disease.

But many people get hyperlipidemia through diets that are heavy in saturated fat and lifestyles that are overloaded with stress situations. Why does stress cause hyperlipidemia? So far, nobody knows for sure—but there is overwhelming evidence that it does. In these instances, the hyperlipidemia is "secondary" to fatty diets and stressful lifestyles.

Lifestyle also includes the taking of drugs: Estrogens, oral contraceptives (the Pill), steroids, and thiazide diuretics are known to cause fat to stick to the artery walls.

But the most tragic victim of hyperlipidemia is the person who eats a diet heavy in saturated fat. His hyperlipidemia is preventable—if only he knew it! Unknowing, he goes right on stuffing himself with saturated fats, condemning his body to illness when it could be healthy and robust.

As described earlier in this chapter, leftover lipids that aren't used as energy are stored in the body, usually settling in the abdomen, thighs and buttocks. When someone says, "That whipped cream went straight to my waistline," or "I loved that chocolate cake so much I'm sitting on it," he isn't kidding. But what's far worse is that the by-products of these foods have found a home in his arteries.

There are five different types of hyperlipidemia. One, Type II, is *primary* or inherited. Although "primary" means that the disease is inherited, most of its victims can still be helped by dietary changes, weight loss and the Institute Formula.

Type I is very rare and is the result of an inherited defect that prevents clearance of chylomicrons from the bloodstream.

Type II is very common and has been divided into two groups. Type IIa patients have abnormally high levels of LDL, while those with Type IIb have too much of both LDL and VLDL.

Type III is fairly rare. Patients with this type of hyperlipidemia cannot convert enough VLDL into LDL. Therefore, they have very high concentrations of both cholesterol and triglyceride in their bloodstreams.

Type IV, as common as Type II, represents a vicious cycle: The triglyceride in VLDL cannot enter the fatty tissues for storage. Therefore, it is carried back to the liver, where it contributes to the production of still more VLDL.

Type V is very rare. It may be inherited, or it may be secondary to another disease (often some type of diabetes). Patients have too much of both chylomicrons and VLDL in their blood.

How Is Hyperlipidemia Detected?

Like another killer, high blood pressure, hyperlipidemia often exists without any noticeable symptoms at all. In many cases, the first indication of it is a heart attack.

Today, many doctors routinely run blood-cholesterol and blood-triglyceride tests on all patients over age 35 or 40. And patients, who know a lot more about fat and its diseases than ever before, often ask for the blood-cholesterol determination. If you do, ask for a triglyceride reading, too; it's also important. Finally, be sure to ask your doctor about the *types* of lipids found in your blood: HDL, LDL, or VLDL. He will probably be surprised to find that you know about the difference, but it's important that you do. If you have high levels of HDL, you are in good shape; but if your levels of LDL and/or VLDL are higher than they should be, you are in trouble *now*, and need to take action to bring those levels down.

There are some signs that make doctors suspect hyperlipidemia, although they don't occur in all, or even most, patients. Severe obesity is often a dead giveaway, since it's almost impossible for a person to be extremely fat without also having elevated cholesterol and triglyceride levels.

Another visible sign is the presence of lumps of hardened fat that collect just under the skin on the elbows, knees, or fingers; in the palms of the hands; or on the eyelids, where they appear as yellowish plaques called xanthomas.

Pain can accompany some cases of hyperlipidemia, but then pain is common to so many diseases that no doctor is going to think of hyperlipidemia first. Still, hyperlipidemic patients can have pain in the legs when walking, soreness of the arms and legs, and occasionally severe abdominal pain. The arm and leg pain result from poor circulation of blood through narrowed arteries, while the abdominal pain often is caused by disorders of the gallbladder (remember, cholesterol was first identified in gallstones).

Worst of all, and most dangerous because it often serves as warning of a heart attack, is a pain in the chest called angina pectoris (some people simply call it angina). Very often, fatal or nonfatal heart attacks begin with this chest pain, which can very easily be confused with indigestion. In fact, about 10 to 20 percent of adults are found to have lost their lives to heart attacks they mistook for indigestion. Coronary heart disease can be silent and lethal—all the more reason for you to actively look for it. Like a burglar, it may be hiding, just waiting for you to get careless.

Diseases to which hyperlipidemia can be secondary include alcoholism, diabetes, pancreatitis (inflammation of the pancreas), hypothyroidism (underfunctioning of the thyroid gland), gallbladder dysfunction and a few exotic diseases that are seldom seen. The presence of these diseases, a family history of any of them, or of severe obesity or heart disease, should lead your doctor to perform blood-cholesterol and triglyceride tests. These will tell not only whether you have hyperlipidemia but, if you do, what type it is.

These tests are simple for you, requiring only the drawing of a blood sample after a twelve- to fourteen-hour fast. If you are taking any of the drugs known to affect blood-lipid levels—estrogens, steroids, birth-control pills, or thiazide diuretics—make sure the doctor knows it. If possible, you should stop taking them for three or four weeks before the blood is drawn.

The blood sample will be sent to a laboratory, where it will be analyzed for cholesterol and triglyceride levels. Although the "normal limits" for cholesterol are listed in medical textbooks as being 150 to 250 milligrams, the warning sign for triglyceride is a reading in excess of 140 milligrams.

When these high levels are found, additional tests will be done to determine the type of hyperlipidemia with which you and your doctor are dealing.

How Is Hyperlipidemia Treated?

Whatever its causes, primary or secondary, the main treatment for hyperlipidemia is a change in diet. The goal is to reduce the dietary intake of cholesterol and saturated fats while at the same time increasing quantities of polyunsaturated fats. Sometimes doctors also use drugs designed to lower the lipid levels. And now we have the Institute Formula—not a drug, but a compound of entirely natural ingredients—to help fight the degenerative diseases that can lead to arteriosclerosis.

In addition to improving the diet and giving the Formula, we also make every effort to improve a hyperlipidemic patient's lifestyle and pattern of exercise. These four elements—diet, the Institute Formula, exercise and lifestyle—together form the Institute Program.

Included in lifestyle, of course, is the elimination (or at least modification) of other factors known to contribute to hyperlipidemia and arteriosclerosis. Excessive use of alcohol and tobacco is one source of blame, and everyone knows it can contribute to many other problems as well as hyperlipidemia. Office jobs can be a harmful factor, and so can inactive leisure hours (better known as laziness), as well as a heavy intake of caffeine in coffee, tea and cola drinks. Sadly, much-beloved chocolate does double duty as a villain, since it contains both saturated fat and caffeine.

If all this sounds like a life of rigid self-sacrifice and discipline, relax. We're not asking you to become teetotalers or to throw aside your office job to become a lumberjack or a ski instructor. But we do encourage you to use moderation: to drink less and exercise more. And even if you do get a lot of exercise, watch out for nightly bouts of beer, pizza and "the tube."

Because each person is different, each Institute Program must be tailored to the individual, to his or her present diet and lifestyle, and to his or her needs in terms of lowering lipid levels. But rarely have we found any person who couldn't benefit from the Institute Program.

Chapter 3

THE PREVENTION BREAKTHROUGH: YOU *CAN* FIGHT BACK

If you've ever visited the Fountain of Youth in St. Augustine, Florida, you probably remember the story the guide tells about why Ponce de Leon thought he was near the source of a magic potion that would keep people young.

De Leon, history tells us, stood five feet three inches tall and came from a fifteenth century society in which life expectancy was about thirty-five years. But when he discovered the land that we now call Florida, he also discovered the Timucuan Indians. What a shock it must have been to find people who stood about six feet tall, were strong and healthy at an age when Europeans were weak and dying, and lived considerably longer!

Perhaps Ponce de Leon was an early nutritionist (or at least on the right track), because he believed that the source of the Indians' height, health and long life lay in what they ate and drank; for some reason we probably will never know, he put most of his faith in the water they drank.

Looking back on that time with the scientific and nutritional knowledge we have today, it's easy to see that Ponce de Leon may not have been too far off. The Timucuan Indians ate mostly the mineral-rich fish they took from the Atlantic Ocean and the vitamin-rich vegetables that grew in the chemical-free soil of that subtropical climate. The water they drank came from a mineral spring that Ponce de Leon thought must be much like the Fountain of Youth he was seeking. (Sadly, he never found the real thing.)

If you visit the Fountain of Youth Park today, the tour guide will give you a drink from that very spring (which is now encased in cement and surrounded by an historical exhibit). You'll notice that the water tastes "funny"—somewhat metallic. That's because it's mineral water. You'll also notice that nothing special happens when you drink it: no puffs of smoke, no flashes of light, no sudden change in your looks or the way you feel, no dramatic loss of ten or fifteen years. But you didn't really expect that, did you?

We all know there are no magic potions. But we also know, after decades of scientific research, that we are not helpless against the aging process. Aging can't be combated with a drink of water, a handful of pills, or a week in an expensive spa—but you can fight back.

The Timucuan Indians drank the water from that mineral spring all their lives, and that's part of the lesson: It takes time to fight time. In order to really protect yourself from degenerative diseases that promote premature aging, you have to maintain good nutritional habits and lifestyles for a long period of time—preferably for life. Obviously, the earlier you start, the more time you'll have to enjoy the benefits. On the other hand, if you wait too long to begin a sound, low-fat, high-nutrition diet, you'll be in trouble. There is a point of no return.

Advanced arteriosclerosis cannot be reversed. After a certain point, your arteries become a virtual graveyard, with the fatty plaques as tombstones. If you wait too long, too long becomes too late.

But how long is too long? It depends. I have already told you that sometimes early and moderate degeneration of the circulation can be stopped and even reversed; if it has not yet started, there are very good chances that it can be prevented.

There's a lot of "maybe" in that paragraph, and it's there for a good reason. What Ponce de Leon didn't know is that there is no such thing as a Fountain of Youth, and no such thing as a sure cure that works the same way for everyone. But there is hope, and it is a very real hope, based on very real and very extensive scientific knowledge.

How do we know that some of the degenerative diseases that lead to arteriosclerosis and heart attack can be stopped, reversed or prevented? To answer that question, I'm going to go backward and tell you how we know that what people eat and drink can get these diseases started in the first place.

Since a complete list of all the evidence and research would fill a whole library, I think a few examples are enough to make the point.

Your Diet and Your Arteries

One of the most dramatic and far-reaching discoveries to come out of the Korean and Vietnam wars had nothing to do with either politics or fighting: It was direct evidence of the influence of dietary fat on the arteries.

The first study to reveal this evidence was done in Korea by William F. Enos, Jr., M.D., and a team of U.S. Army pathologists, who performed autopsies on 300 American soldiers who had lost their lives. In particular, they examined the coronary arteries of these unfortunate victims of war, most of whom were very young—between 18 and 28 years of age.

The pathologists found that 77 percent of the American soldiers (who had eaten typically high-fat American diets all their lives) already had fatty deposits of cholesterol and other lipids in their coronary arteries, as evidenced by fatty streaks, fatty plaques and actual atherosclerotic narrowing of the coronary arteries. But when, in a later study, they examined 114 Japanese (whose Oriental diets had been very low in saturated fat), only about 2 percent had the same evidence of beginning degenerative disease. The difference between 77 percent and 2 percent was astounding—Dr. Enos and his colleagues were thunderstruck! Years later, similar teams of U.S. Army pathologists found almost exactly the same differences between American and Vietnamese soldiers killed in Vietnam.

Of course, careful scientists immediately raised the question: What about racial differences between the Caucasians (Americans) and Orientals (Japanese and Vietnamese)? Couldn't these have been responsible instead of their diets?

Of the many investigators who tried to answer this critical question, one of the first was Ancel Keys, Ph.D., of the University of Minnesota. He and his team studied the diets, particularly the saturated-fat intakes, of many countries in Europe and the Orient, and compared them to the diets and saturated-fat intakes of people from the same countries who had emigrated to America. Going back several generations, they then compared the death rates from arteriosclerotic diseases in the same people.

The distinctions were very clear-cut. Oriental diets, in particular, are very low in saturated fat; the death rates from coronary heart disease are very low in China, Japan and the other countries of that region, and they stay low as long as the people stay in the Orient and consume those low-fat diets.

But members of Oriental families who moved to America and started eating our high-saturated-fat diet started to show changes even in the first generation. In the second generation, increases in their lipid and cholesterol levels became greater, and so did their death rates from arteriosclerotic disease. By the third generation, the lipid and cholesterol levels—and the death rates—were the same as those of Americans whose families had been here right from the beginning of our country!

The young American soldiers, it seemed, had shown signs of early arteriosclerosis because of their fatty diets, not because of racial differences between Caucasians and Orientals.

The evidence was so strong, and the soldiers were so young, that it made scientists wonder just when arteriosclerosis starts. To find out, many investigators ran studies on the arteries of children who had been killed in accidents. And the frightening but overwhelming evidence showed that the fatty streaks of beginning arteriosclerotic deposits begin in early childhood—heavy streaks and deposits were found in the arteries of children as young as 7, 8 and 9 years old.

In about half of the American population, these degenerative deposits grow as the child grows, until the inevitable occurs: The child becomes an adult with advanced arteriosclerosis, suffers from premature signs of aging and dies an early death from heart attack or stroke.

The Fat of the Land

Dr. Keys also did studies in Europe that reinforced his belief in the connection between dietary saturated fat and heart disease. In Italy, for example, he found that a province near Bologna was famous for its rich, fatty food—pork, butter, eggs, pasta made with eggs, lots of cream sauces and butter-rich pastries—and also had a very high rate of coronary heart disease. But in a nearby province in the same country, the people had developed recipes that were low in saturated fats and high in polyunsaturated fats, and in that province the rate of death from coronary heart disease was very low.

When these studies were extended to children, the results showed even more clearly how important diet is, and how much your health can be affected by where you are born and grow up.

Babies, it turns out, have just about the same blood-lipid levels no matter where they are born or what race they are. If someone showed you a set of infant arteries and asked, "Where was this baby born?" you wouldn't have a clue.

But if you saw a set of arteries from 5-, 6-, 7-, or 8-year-olds (or older children), you still wouldn't be able to pinpoint the country, but you'd have a pretty good chance of guessing the part of the world. Children from regions favoring a low-fat diet have relatively clear arteries and low blood-cholesterol levels. But American children, and those from other Western countries in which high-fat diets are popular, have fat-streaked arteries and much higher blood-cholesterol levels.

Clearly, we're not doing our youngsters any favors when we feed them bacon and eggs every morning, tell them whole milk is "nature's best food" (they should be drinking low-fat or non-fat milk), and let them eat junk food filled with fat. Fortunately, when they're very young, it's easy to undo the damage in most cases. (There are cases of childhood arteriosclerosis, heart attack and stroke on record, but they are very rare and are caused by inherited defects and diseases, not by diet.)

Dr. Keys and hundreds of other researchers (far too many to be listed here) have now done the same kinds of studies of both children and adults in many other countries, including England, Scotland, France, Finland, West Germany and even the Soviet Union. The results are too obvious to be ignored, even by skeptics: Where there's a lot of saturated fat in the diet, there's coronary heart disease.

My Personal Experience

My own evidence of the relationship between saturated fat and degenerative diseases came almost by accident. I call it serendipity: the lucky discovery of one thing when you've been looking for something else.

I was investigating diseases of the liver back in the early 30s, and trying to learn what effects heavy doses of saturated fat would have on that organ; in particular, I suspected that fatty diets had a lot to do with cirrhosis of the liver. I was working with laboratory rats and other experimental animals, and I have to tell you that I had my share of trouble: The animals were too smart to eat great gobs of fat willingly, and I had to force-feed them.

When I examined the dead animals to see what the fat had done to their livers, I made a surprising discovery. Heavy deposits of fat had clogged their arteries, especially at the junctions where two arteries came together or branched off in different directions. Arteriosclerotic plaques were all over those arteries, and the insides were obviously narrowed.

When I examined other animals who had not been given the fatty diets, I found almost no plaques and narrowing at all. What stronger evidence could a research scientist ask for?

When I turned my studies from liver disease to heart disease, I used fatty diets to create arteriosclerosis in experimental animals so that I could try out different ways of curing it. If you ask me how I know that saturated fat contributes to arteriosclerosis, heart disease and stroke, I'll say, "Easy! I've made it happen." Much more important was learning how to make it *stop*.

The First Step

If the drain in your sink is clogged with grease and garbage, the most effective way to open it is to call the Roto-Rooter man and have him ream it out. But you can't Roto-Rooter an artery. Human tissue is far more delicate than iron pipes and couldn't stand the rough scraping it would take to get rid of nature's grease and garbage, the arteriosclerotic plaques.

Next best for your drain is a caustic substance such as lye, which you pour down in the form of Drano or Liquid Plumber. But arteries can't take lye, either. Many drugs have been formulated that will *partially* dissolve arteriosclerotic plaques, but they work very slowly and can't do a thorough job—and some of them have very unpleasant and even dangerous side effects.

The *easiest* way to have a clear drain, of course, is not to pour all that grease and garbage down there in the first place. So it is with arteries: The easiest way is prevention.

The Preventive Balance

I've already told you that you can't live without lipids, and you can't live (at least not very long or very well) with too much of them. Now I'm going to tell you that you can't live with too few of them, either.

It has already been established that obesity, high-saturated-fat diets and high levels of blood lipids (especially LDL and VLDL) are dangerous and contribute to coronary heart disease. More recently, scientists have learned that *under-*

weight, super-low-fat diets, and very low levels of blood lipids are also dangerous; people with these problems don't usually die of heart attacks, but they have very high rates of death from other diseases, such as tuberculosis and cancer.

The answer, therefore, is *balance*. You shouldn't overdo your lipid intake, but you shouldn't under-do it, either. And you have to balance the amount of HDL against the amount of LDL to get a favorable ratio. If you put the right amounts of the right kinds of lipids into your body, the body will put them to good use.

The way your body puts lipids to use—or allows them to abuse it—is determined by the function called "metabolism." Metabolism is a food processor that makes a Cuisinart look like a Tinker Toy; it's extremely complicated, but how well it works depends on what you give it to work with.

Your metabolism processes everything you eat and drink, breaks it down into all its usable elements and distributes those elements to the different parts of the body, eliminating useless materials as waste. But there's a hitch. As you know, even LDL is not useless—in the right amounts it is needed to produce energy. Your metabolism, however, has no more intelligence than your Cuisinart. It can't tell the difference between the right and wrong kinds and amounts of lipids. You have to do the thinking for it.

You have to decide what to put into your food processor and what to leave out. And that's not an easy decision, because everyone is different. What's right for you may be wrong for someone else. I'm going to help you learn how to make the decision wisely, based on a personal assessment of your individual needs.

The Coronary Risk Factors

How can you assess your individual needs? By evaluating your "coronary risk factors." These are characteristics that almost all doctors agree place a person in danger of arteriosclerosis, heart attack and stroke. The more risk factors you have, the worse off you are.

But you can still fight back. While there are some risk factors labeled "uncontrollable" because there's nothing you can do about them, there are more that are controllable. These you can change—and if you can change enough of them in the right way, you should be able to *decrease* your chances of having coronary heart disease and *increase* your chances of having a healthier, longer life.

The *uncontrollable risk factors* are:

1. Your sex (males are at greater risk than females)
2. Your age (the younger you are, the less the damage already done, and the more time you have to change your controllable risk factors)
3. Your place of birth and growing up (you can't change the diet you were fed as a child, but you can change what you're eating now)
4. Your heredity (you can't change the traits you inherited, but you can do something to counteract the bad ones)

The *controllable risk factors* are:

1. Your diet (controlled by you)
2. Your weight (controlled by your diet)
3. Your blood-lipid levels (affected by your diet)
4. Your blood pressure (affected by your diet and, if necessary, by medical treatment)
5. Your activity (the more appropriate exercise you get, the less your risk)
6. Your lifestyle (the better you can learn to handle stress, the less your risk)
7. Your habits (smoking, heavy alcohol drinking, and using certain drugs all increase your risk)

It's comforting to know that the controllable risk factors outnumber the uncontrollable ones. And the news gets even better: Even though you can't change the uncontrollable factors, you *can* change some of their effects.

1. *Your sex:* If you are a man, you can reduce that risk factor by taking the Institute Formula and carefully following the dietary, exercise, and lifestyle plans of the Institute Program. If you are a woman, you may not have to be quite as strict as the men.
2. *Your age:* No matter how old you are, if you do not already have advanced arteriosclerosis and irreversible damage to the heart you can benefit by starting the Institute Program *now*.

3. *Your place of birth and growing up:* If you were born and raised in a country where the diet is high in saturated fat (for example, the United States), you can start repairing the damage with the Institute Program.
4. *Your heredity:* If you inherited a tendency toward high blood-lipid levels and coronary heart disease, you can lessen your chances of following that tendency to its debilitating or fatal end.

Obviously, nobody needs to tell you where you stand regarding the first three uncontrollable risk factors. But what about the fourth? Just how important is heredity in the pattern of arteriosclerosis, heart disease and stroke?

It's *very* important. You may have inherited one of the hereditary types of hyperlipidemia described in chapter 2. But how do you know? And just how much difference does it make, anyway?

The Two Faces of Lipoproteins

Actually there are *four* kinds of lipoproteins, as described in chapter 2, but two of them stand out as the most important factors in the creation of arteriosclerosis. They are LDL, which causes fats to stay in the body and stick to the insides of arteries, and HDL, which is the "detergent" lipoprotein that helps to rid the body of harmful fat deposits.

This concept of LDL and HDL is an accepted scientific principle. I think the innumerable research papers that went into reaching it were summed up very nicely by Simeon Margolis, M.D., Ph.D., of the Johns Hopkins School of Medicine, when he wrote in April, 1981:

> *Levels of serum cholesterol, carried mainly on low-density lipoproteins (LDL), correlate strongly with the development of myocardial infarction [heart attack]. In contrast, considerable evidence indicates that high-density lipoprotein (HDL) protects against coronary heart disease.*

To put it very bluntly, LDL is the killer and HDL is the saver. Fortunately, HDL has some helpers.

Your body is made up of more than 1,000 trillion cells. Nobody knows exactly how many because it's impossible to count them. The body is a universe in itself, almost limitless. But it's not defenseless. It has many defense mechanisms; prob-

ably the best known is its ability to form antibodies that help
you to fight off infections. Another is the presence of an army
of protectors called "LDL receptors" because they *receive* the
LDL from your blood.

If you think 1,000 trillion is a huge number, consider this:
There are approximately 25,000 to 40,000 LDL receptors for each
of those cells. The LDL receptors "sit" around the outside of
the cell like Secret Service agents guarding the President. When
faced with an attack of LDL, the receptors *grab* the LDL (actually, they soak it out of the blood like sponges), absorb it,
metabolize it and pass it on into the cell to be used in the
production of energy. If your LDL receptors are working well,
most of the LDL in your blood will be captured and put to work
where it can do you some good.

Unfortunately, some people don't have enough LDL receptors to do their job, or the ones they do have are defective
and allow a lot of LDL to escape and form atherosclerotic plaques
that stick to the insides of their arteries. LDL-receptor deficiency
runs in families, and members of those families are in great
danger of developing arteriosclerosis, heart attacks and strokes.
The lack of enough LDL receptors is seen in Type II hyperlipidemia, described in chapter 2.

That's a good example of uncontrollable risk factor number 4. There is no way you can change who your mother and
father were, or the genetic legacy they passed on to you. But
if you do have a lack of LDL receptors, or any other inherited
inability to handle the lipids in your blood, the Institute Formula
can help you.

The Institute Formula is not a bottle full of LDL receptors.
(I'll tell you exactly what's in it in chapters 4 and 5.) It is a
combination of naturally occurring ingredients that have been
shown to do the job the LDL receptors would do if they were
there—or if there were enough of them. The Institute Formula
is a kind of replacement therapy: It makes up for something
that's lacking.

What if you already have enough LDL receptors? Then
the Institute Formula will help them to be more efficient and
effective.

Either way, you can't lose. If heredity has dealt you a
bad hand, the Institute Formula will give you a better chance
of beating the odds. If you already have a good hand, the
Formula will make it even better. Since you are not competing
against another person, but only against degenerative disease,
the best hand you can get is likely to make you a winner.

The Story of Lisa and Julie

How do I know that Type II hyperlipidemia can be helped? Let me tell you a story from my own experience, a story with a tragic beginning but a very happy ending.

Lisa was a 13-year-old girl who had inherited a lot of wonderful characteristics from her parents, grandparents and other ancestors. She was intelligent, pretty, energetic and well coordinated, and even blessed with musical talent. Unfortunately, she also inherited Type II hyperlipidemia.

Lisa lived with her mother and younger brother; her father had died several years before of a heart attack, even though he was only 30 years old and apparently in excellent health. He had been proud that, aside from the usual childhood diseases, he had "never had a sick day in his life." When the sudden and unexpected heart attack ended his short life, his family's astonishment was almost as great as their grief.

One night, Lisa was awakened by a sharp pain in her chest, just below the breastbone. The pain radiated down her left arm, into her back, and up the left side of her neck and jaw. She felt dizzy, broke into a drenching sweat, grew cold and clammy, became nauseated and threw up.

Awakened by her child's cries, Lisa's mother rushed into the room and found the girl weak, pale and "white as a ghost." She immediately called the fire department, which sent its emergency paramedic ambulance. As the vehicle rushed Lisa to the hospital with screaming sirens, the paramedics did everything they could do to revive the little girl who had become unconscious, stopped breathing and appeared to be lifeless. But they couldn't do enough. When they reached the emergency room, the tragic diagnosis was "DOA"—Dead On Arrival.

What could have struck such a young, apparently healthy child? There was no time to find out then, because Lisa's mother, Julie, had collapsed. Like her daughter, she was pale, perspiring freely, chilled and clammy. The emergency room doctor felt for her pulse, but couldn't find it.

Immediately, the resuscitation team placed an electroshock machine on Julie's chest. In response to the shock, her chest heaved, and her heart resumed its beating. With oxygen and intravenous fluids the doctors were slowly able to revive her, but it was obvious that she had been suffering from more than the shock of her daughter's death.

An electrocardiogram taken in the emergency room revealed a classic massive myocardial infarction—an almost fatal heart attack. And Julie was only 35 years old.

Later, as Julie recovered in the hospital, her doctors found that her blood cholesterol level was almost 2,000 milligrams (the normal level for her age is 200 milligrams). She also had, on her knuckles, elbows and heels, the classic fatty lumps called xanthoma that are so often seen in cases of hereditary hyperlipidemia.

Meanwhile, the coroner's office had performed an autopsy on Lisa's body and found that the cause of death had been advanced arteriosclerosis of all the coronary arteries, with complete obstruction of the left main artery of the heart. The arteries of this 13-year-old girl looked worse than those of most elderly people who die of heart attacks and arteriosclerosis! Also, xanthomas were found on her knuckles, elbows and heels; her condition was nearly a carbon copy of her mother's. Examination showed that the lumps were almost solid cholesterol.

These findings led the doctors to make a diagnosis of Type II hyperlipidemia for both mother and daughter—that is, hereditary inability to metabolize LDL. But what of Lisa's brother?

When his blood was examined, the condition of the 9-year-old boy was found to be normal in all respects: cholesterol level (165 milligrams), electrocardiogram, blood chemistry, everything—including knuckles, elbows and heels free of xanthomas.

This was not surprising to the doctors, who knew that hereditary diseases strike some family members and skip others altogether. If you study the laws of inheritance put forth by the Austrian monk Gregor Mendel more than a hundred years ago, you learn that there are definite patterns. You can predict pretty closely how many members of a family will have certain characteristics, such as brown hair, blue eyes, freckles, tallness or shortness, excellent or poor singing voices, as well as minor or life-threatening diseases. Lisa's brother was one of the lucky ones the Type II hyperlipidemia skipped; Lisa, obviously, was not.

Looking back into the families of both Julie and her husband, the doctors found that Julie's mother had atherosclerosis of the legs, and her father was being treated for the aftermath of a stroke. Her husband's parents had both suffered from heart disease and high blood pressure. It was almost inevitable that at least one of this couple's children would die of heart disease, probably early in life.

But I told you the story had a happy ending. The family certainly deserved it, after all the tragedy they had been through.

Even so, it wasn't very likely. Considering the circumstances, no one expected Julie to live very long, and it looked as though her 9-year-old son would soon be left an orphan.

Julie had two huge strikes against her: first, her inherited Type II hyperlipidemia (an uncontrollable risk factor), and second, the American diet, heavy in saturated fats, that she had been eating all her life (a *controllable* risk factor). We hadn't come to strike three (a fatal heart attack), and we were determined not to.

Many people contributed a great deal of time and effort to keeping Julie alive, not the least of whom was a psychiatrist who helped her cope with the terrible tragedies she had been through and regain her will to live. Among those who helped Julie survive was a team of dietitians who had worked with me in 1945 when I first developed my low-fat, low-cholesterol diet. In addition, a group of my fellow physicians at Los Angeles General Hospital accepted the challenge of Julie's case and gave her carefully regulated doses of cholesterol-lowering agents, such as soya phosphatidyl choline and inositol with soya lecithin (more about these later). Added to these were agents known as ion-exchange resins, substances derived from the bark of trees. These resins are not absorbed by the body, but move through the bowel, sucking up lipids and cholesterol before passing out of the body; they are cleansing agents.

Supplementing these measures, we began an exercise program for Julie as soon as she was well enough to handle it. She stayed for some time in a rehabilitation hospital, where she followed the diet created for her, exercised more and more as she got better and better, took the dietary supplements planned for her, and stayed away from cigarettes and alcoholic beverages. The xanthomas on her knuckles, elbows and heels gradually shrank and eventually disappeared, and her blood-cholesterol level moved slowly downward until it reached a healthy level and remained there. Little by little, her emotional outlook improved, and that of course reduced the stress of the grief she had been suffering. Instead of dying of a heart attack as expected, Julie recovered.

For how long? I don't know, because the story isn't over yet. This case history began more than fifteen years ago; Julie is now in her fifties, remarried, and living in another part of the country. Occasionally we hear from her, and the reward of knowing how well she's doing is more than worth all the time and hard work that went into our fight against her disease.

The case of Lisa and Julie is only one of many experiences

I've had with both primary and secondary hyperlipidemia, and I am only one of many doctors who have been fortunate enough to experience the rewards of successful treatment. We *know* that diets and food supplements can have beneficial effects on hyperlipidemia—even the inherited types. How do we know it? Easy! We've made it happen.

Your Personal Profile

Fortunately, cases such as that of Lisa and Julie are not very common. But having normal, healthy LDL receptors is no guarantee against an invasion of LDL or the formation of arteriosclerotic plaques. Even the best protectors can be overwhelmed. If you overload your bloodstream with dietary saturated fats, that's just what you're doing: overwhelming your LDL receptors with more lipids than they can handle.

Whether you have inherited high levels of LDL or have done yourself in with a fatty diet, help is available, and the goal is the same: to achieve a *good* balance of HDL and LDL in your system.

Of course, if you are young, slim and feeling fine, you may think you are already home free. Why interfere with good health? The fatty American diet is the reason. If you love hot dogs, ham and eggs, steak, French fries, grilled cheese sandwiches, butter cookies, Hershey bars, ice cream and apple pie (and what American doesn't?), your happy state of youth, slimness and well being will not last long. It won't change overnight, but gradually that state will become one of premature age, overweight and misery. No matter what condition you're in now, there's always room for improvement.

It's the *degree* of improvement that makes the difference between you and somebody else. Do you have to correct an existing problem, or just prevent a future one? Do you have to lose fifty pounds? Thirty? Fifteen? None? Do you already watch your fat intake, or are you addicted to barbequed ribs and chocolate eclairs? Do you spend your free time watching TV, or playing tennis? Are you "cool," or do you flash a hot temper you later regret?

All these conditions have a lot to do with your chances of having arteriosclerosis, and with the kinds of changes you'll have to make to prevent it. To determine the changes that are right for you, you have to take several good, long looks at yourself.

Look at Your Family Tree

What are the chances that you have inherited a type of hyperlipidemia? To find out, you have to look backward.

Take out your family album and look at all the relatives pictured there. Have a pencil and paper handy so that you can make notes and get a clear idea of your family's health history.

First of all, consider your parents. Did (or does) either of them have a heart attack, stroke, chest pains or any other sign of atherosclerosis? What were (or are) their weight classifications: thin, normal, a little overweight, or downright fat?

Grandparents are also important, on both sides of the family—and so are aunts and uncles, great aunts and uncles, cousins and even your brothers and sisters. All the members of your family have places in the Mendelian law of heredity, and their physical traits and conditions are determined according to different patterns. These patterns change every time a member of your family marries someone from another family and they have a child; then a whole new set of patterns is added. This is why you have to look at both sides of the family to learn which diseases occur often, occasionally, or not at all.

With the help of the family album try to remember: If a certain member of the family is now dead, how did he or she die? For those who are still living, what diseases have affected their lives? Have any of them had heart trouble? Have any of them had strokes? Do any of them suffer from high blood pressure or the chest pains known as angina pectoris? This will help you to understand whether or not you are in a risky position—whether there is a strong, medium or mild chance that you, too, will experience a heart attack, stroke or any of the other degenerative results of atherosclerosis.

How many heart-diseased relatives does it take to make you a high risk? There are no definite numbers. The situation is not black and white. There is not one set of people with familial hyperlipidemia and another set without it. There is a very large gray area in between.

It's possible that you may have mixed genes. One member of your family, say a grandparent or an uncle, may pass on a gene that skips most members of the family except one. This is a recessive trait, just like blue eyes. Just one case of hyperlipidemia may occur in a family in which most members have received the genes of the long-lived ancestors. But if many family members have died or suffered from heart disease and its complications, your chances of having these problems are greater than if no relatives or very few had heart trouble.

Now that you have evaluated your family history, you have the answers to one of the first questions you will be asked by a doctor. And that is where you have to go to find out for sure whether you are lacking in LDL receptors or whether your blood-lipid level is low, normal or high: to a doctor. Tell him you want to know where you stand as a cardiac risk, and be sure to request not only a blood-cholesterol test but an evaluation of the triglycerides and the *types* of lipoproteins in your blood.

The doctor will take a blood sample for testing, and ask about your family history (if he doesn't already know it). He will weigh you and ask how many cigarettes you smoke and how much alcohol you drink. He will take your blood pressure. If he isn't your lifelong family doctor and doesn't know you well, he may test your blood for sugar as well as lipids, to see whether you are one of the many "hidden" diabetics.

All these factors will be considered—and if your doctor is on the staff of a large hospital or has access to sophisticated equipment, he may feed the information to a computer that can weigh all the possibilities and make a very educated prediction as to just how long you can be expected to live!

Of course, these computers are not psychics or clairvoyants. They can make predictions based on probabilities, which are in turn based upon facts about you, your family and the lipid content of your blood. But they can't predict whether you'll be bitten by a rabid dog while jogging. This is science, after all, not fortune-telling.

The prediction will tell you approximately how much longer you can expect to live in your present condition, but by now you know that you have the power to change that prediction in your favor.

If you find that you do not have a strong inherited risk, you may consider yourself very lucky, indeed. But you are still not safe; you have to consider all those controllable risk factors. You know that a fatty diet, lack of exercise, stress, smoking and too much drinking can bring about clogging of the arteries even in the healthiest and lowest-risk people.

If you are already a low-risk person, why, you may wonder, should you bother with the Institute Program? You should follow it as a preventive measure against future deterioration and as "insurance" to keep you in the low-risk category. In these cases, the Program may not increase your life span, since it's probably already about as long as anyone's can be expected to be—the same as it was at the time of your birth.

On the other hand, if you are free of bad genes but have thrown a monkey wrench into your own works by eating foods heavy in saturated fats, smoking, drinking heavily, being inactive, and living under great stress, these bad habits have probably shortened the life span that was genetically predicted for you at birth. If you can stop your harmful behavior in time and reverse the process of deterioration, you may be able to bring that predicted life span back to or close to its original long length.

The Institute Program can help you reduce the risk of death from the controllable risk factors. At the same time, you'll find that it increases your health and well being, as well as the functioning of your metabolism—the way your body processes the food you eat and makes it work either for you or against you.

I realize that there are many people who simply will not go to see a doctor unless they are seriously ill or in great pain. If you are one of those, you can still get a fairly good general idea of where you stand as a coronary risk. Evaluate the four uncontrollable risk factors. Then take a look at the controllable risk factors to see what you can do to improve your position.

Look at Your Weight

It's not easy to admit you're overweight, unless it's so obvious you can't ignore it. Then you make jokes about having your clothes made by Omar the Tent Maker, and laugh to pretend it doesn't hurt. But it does, physically as well as emotionally.

It hurts you physically even if you're only a little bit overweight. Why should a few pounds hurt? Because they're a beginning. They are like a few innocent little dandelion seeds— ignore them and the first thing you know, your lawn is covered with weeds, and they're choking out the grass. In the same way, those few pounds equal a few arteriosclerotic plaques that are on their way to choking your arteries.

If you're a beanpole, you probably think you have nothing to worry about. Think again. As I mentioned earlier, being underweight is dangerous, too. When the Council on Epidemiology of the American Heart Association held its annual conference in Washington, D.C., in March of 1981, three different groups of research scientists reported on the dangers of being underweight, agreeing that "low relative dietary fat, low body weight, and low serum cholesterol are associated with excess mortality due to causes *other* than coronary heart disease" (italics mine). The famous Framingham study of heart disease reports that men with lower than normal blood-cholesterol levels are three times more likely to develop cancer of the colon than are men with normal cholesterol readings.

Once again, the answer is *balance*. The doctors at the Council on Epidemiology conference agreed that "mortality increased as levels of LDL increased, but decreased with increasing ratio of HDL to LDL." Moreover, the Heart Association recommends that, in general, normal people should consume about 30 to 35 percent of their total calorie intake as fat—the right kind of fat: polyunsaturated.

Note the description "normal" people. That's why your Personal Profile is so important. If you have hyperlipidemia, if you are overweight, or if you are underweight, you are not "normal." Being normal is your goal. The kind of diet that is right for you will depend on the results of your Personal Profile. (Remember, you may look and feel normal and still have hyperlipidemia. That's why, at the risk of being repetitious, I'm going to urge you again to see a doctor and have your blood lipids tested.)

How much should you weigh? If you're not *grossly* overweight or underweight, how can you tell what weight will promote good health?

Look at the table of desirable weights for men and women provided by the Metropolitan Life Insurance Company. You've probably seen it before; for about twenty-five years it has been published and republished in newspapers, books and magazines all over the world. The table has lasted so long and gotten such heavy coverage because it is a good general guideline for weight, and it can be trusted.

You can see that the table doesn't give you a specific number as your ideal weight, but a range. That's because it's impossible for anyone to reach a specific weight and stick to it. Your weight changes a little bit from day to day, and even within the hours of a single day. As long as it doesn't go steadily up or steadily down, but stays within the range that's ideal for your sex, age and body build, you're in good shape.

Because your weight changes during the day, you should weigh yourself at the same time and under the same conditions. You'll probably notice that your weight will be just a little bit different each day. But it isn't necessary to weigh yourself every

DESIRABLE WEIGHTS FOR MEN AND WOMEN
According to Height and Frame, Ages 25 and Over

HEIGHT (in shoes)*	WEIGHT IN POUNDS (in indoor clothing)		
	Small Frame	Medium Frame	Large Frame
MEN			
5' 2"	112–120	118–129	126–141
3"	115–123	121–133	129–144
4"	118–126	124–136	132–148
5"	121–129	127–139	135–152
6"	124–133	130–143	138–156
7"	128–137	134–147	142–161
8"	132–141	138–152	147–166
9"	136–145	142–156	151–170
10"	140–150	146–160	155–174
11"	144–154	150–165	159–179
6' 0"	148–158	154–170	164–184
1"	152–162	158–175	168–189
2"	156–167	162–180	173–194
3"	160–171	167–185	178–199
4"	164–175	172–190	182–204
WOMEN			
4'10"	92– 98	96–107	104–119
11"	94–101	98–110	106–122
5' 0"	96–104	101–113	109–125
1"	99–107	104–116	112–128
2"	102–110	107–119	115–131
3"	105–113	110–122	118–134
4"	108–116	113–126	121–138
5"	111–119	116–130	125–142
6"	114–123	120–135	129–146
7"	118–127	124–139	133–150
8"	122–131	128–143	137–154
9"	126–135	132–147	141–158
10"	130–140	136–151	145–163
11"	134–144	140–155	149–168
6' 0"	138–148	144–159	153–173

SOURCE: Reprinted with special permission from *Statistical Bulletin*, Metropolitan Life Insurance Company, October, 1977, p. 5.
NOTE: Prepared by the Metropolitan Life Insurance Company. Derived primarily from data of the *Build and Blood Pressure Study, 1959*, Society of Actuaries.
*1-inch heels for men and 2-inch heels for women.

day—and if you are on a weight-changing program it can be very discouraging to see these daily changes. If they don't change enough, you may become depressed and think your diet is worthless. If they change in the wrong direction, you may throw your hands up and give up altogether.

So forget about a daily routine. Weigh yourself once a week—for example, every Monday morning. If you're on a weight-changing program, keep a record of how much you have lost or gained each week. Don't expect giant steps. Sudden losses or gains of weight are dangerous, which is only one reason you should stay away from fad diets, gimmicks and pills that promise to take off (or add) maxi-pounds in mini-time. The most you can lose or gain safely is about two or three pounds a week. It's slow, but it's worth it. While pounds are slowly dropping off or adding on, your arteries are shaping up, too.

Look at Your Diet

What kinds of foods are you eating now? What kinds of foods do you like? A quick look in your refrigerator and pantry will give you an idea of the kinds of changes you're going to have to make to take good care of your arteries.

Is the refrigerator loaded with eggs, bacon, butter, cheese, mayonnaise, whole milk, cream, whipped cream, sour cream, and the like? Do your pantry shelves reveal tins of creamed soup, pancake mix, chocolate, cookies, shrimp, noodles, caviar, potato chips, cheese crackers and cake mixes? These spell Trouble.

On the other hand, if you find fresh fruits and vegetables, fish, very lean meat, low-fat milk, clear soups, wheat bread, grain cereals and snacks such as wheat crackers, walnuts and toasted soybeans, you are already well on the way to a healthy low-fat diet.

Do you really have to give up all those luscious high-fat foods? Not necessarily. It depends on both your blood-lipid level and your weight. If you do *not* have familial hyperlipidemia, and if your weight is *normal*, you can safely eat those foods in *moderation*. Your doctor will have to advise you about your lipid level after taking a blood sample. As for your weight, if you're on a reducing program, hold one or two goodies out as an occasional reward for reaching a goal. Eating them only once in a while will make them "extra special" and you'll enjoy them even more—partly because they are rare treats, and partly because you know you are doing yourself so much good by limiting them to once in a while.

Look at Your Cookbooks

Pick a cookbook from the shelf at random. Open it to any page at random. Run your finger down the list of ingredients for any recipe at random. I'd be willing to bet that you'll find at least three ingredients that are loaded with saturated fat. Look at this one for example:

CRAB MEAT CHIP DIP

1 cup *crab meat*	⅛ teaspoon garlic powder
¼ cup lemon juice	2 dashes red pepper
1 3-ounce package *cream cheese*	1 teaspoon Worcestershire sauce
¼ cup *heavy cream*	½ teaspoon salt
2 tablespoons *mayonnaise*	⅛ teaspoon MSG
1 teaspoon minced onion	

Combine all ingredients. Serve as a dip for *potato chips.*

And that's only an *appetizer!* (I admit, I had to turn the pages once to find that one. The first recipe I looked at had only two high-saturated-fat ingredients: ¼ cup butter and 1 pound ground chuck.)

But if you make a spot check of most cookbooks (not counting those that are specifically devoted to low-calorie or low-fat recipes), you'll find that the majority of ingredient lists are loaded with saturated fat. That's characteristic of the American diet.

What can you do about it? Give up all those delicious but damaging foods and live on bean sprouts, wheat germ and papaya juice? Of course not. Nothing that extreme is good for you; you need a certain amount of fat to remain healthy.

What you *can* do about it is make some changes in the way you cook as well as in the foods you use. Believe it or not, some of the most elaborate gourmet recipes can be deprived of their high saturated-fat content and still be rich, creamy and out of this world in taste.

Take that crab meat dip, for instance. The first ingredient, crab meat, is a shellfish, high in cholesterol. Nothing that isn't also a shellfish is an adequate taste substitute for crab meat. So don't try to change it. You know your diet needs some cholesterol, so let this be it—and reserve the recipe for once in a while instead of often.

Next we come to cream cheese. That's a cholesterol blockbuster, since there's saturated fat in both the cheese and the cream that's added to it. What can you do? Easy. Substitute

3 ounces of low-fat cottage cheese into which you have mixed 1 tablespoon of low-fat dry milk powder.

As a substitute for the heavy cream, stir 1 tablespoon of low-fat milk powder into ¼ cup of low-fat milk (commercial skim milk or low-fat milk powder you have already mixed with water according to package directions). The milk powder, by the way, is loaded with vitamins and other nutrients as well as being low in fat.

The next ingredient, mayonnaise, is made with egg yolks and oil. You have two choices: Substitute low-fat yogurt (this, of course, will change the taste considerably), or use low-fat mayonnaise.

When you have mixed all these ingredients together and chilled the mixture, serve it with wheat crackers instead of potato chips (you have no idea *what* they've been fried in!). *Voilà!* A beautiful "chip" dip, delicious, healthy and low in saturated fat.

Now that you have the idea, it can be a lot of fun going through your cookbooks and making changes. First of all, take a pencil and every time you see the word "butter," scratch it out and write in "polyunsaturated margarine." Wherever you find an ingredient high in saturated fat, insert a low-fat replacement. Low-fat yogurt is a natural substitute for sour cream. Olive oil is easily replaced by safflower or soy oil. And if you make cream soups with an extra-rich mixture of low-fat milk and milk powder, I seriously doubt that *anyone* will be able to tell the difference.

What about eggs? There really is no substitute for a fried egg. But there are several substitutes for scrambled eggs, omelets and the eggs you use as a binder in meat loaves and pastries. Egg substitutes usually come frozen in a carton (the same size as a cream carton), and can be found in the frozen-food departments of most supermarkets. They look like scrambled eggs before they're cooked, but they contain no yolks and no cholesterol. When cooked, they look and taste like scrambled eggs. By following the directions on the package, you can use egg substitutes in baking and in making meat loaf, just as if you were using real eggs. It works! And you can live without fried eggs, can't you?

You can't? Have your blood-lipid level checked. If it is not already above the upper limit (only a doctor can tell you that), then you *can* have real eggs—even fried. Just limit them to two a week (which makes them a special treat), and cook them in polyunsaturated margarine instead of butter or (even worse!) bacon grease.

If your blood-lipid level is over the limit, you may *have* to learn to live without fried eggs—and a lot of other foods, too. But check with your doctor before you start feeling deprived. And if you do have to give up fried eggs, try cooking egg *whites;* it's only the yolk that contains cholesterol. Scrambled egg whites are a personal favorite of mine, and a clever cook can do wonders with them.

These are just hints to get you started. If you enjoy cooking, you'll have a lot of fun changing recipes and being creative. If you don't enjoy cooking, just make a few basic changes in your routine shopping list; polyunsaturated margarine for butter, skim milk for whole milk, and so on. And if somebody else cooks for you, tie a ribbon around this book and make a gift of it!

Reducing your intake of calories is another matter. Saturated and polyunsaturated oils are exactly the same in calories, and so are butter and polyunsaturated margarine. If you are overweight, you will have to make some sacrifices in order to get back to normal—but you still won't have to give up everything you like.

Look at Your Pots and Pans

If you use cooking utensils that cause food to stick, you may be getting a lot of exercise washing dishes and scouring pans, but you probably also use large quantities of butter and lard in an effort to prevent sticking. However, if you use nonstick pans, you can eliminate the fat and calories that exist in lubricating agents, and find a more enjoyable way to exercise your arms.

Of course, entire sets of new pots and pans can be pretty expensive, especially in these days of inflation. If you can't or don't want to spend that much money all at once, make the changeover a little at a time. Buy one nonstick pan, and throw the old pan away. Do the same again as soon as you can. Eventually you will have a complete set of nonstick cookware; in the meantime, use polyunsaturated margarine and cooking oils to keep food from sticking to your old pots and pans.

You can also do a lot of cooking without any fat at all. Roast meats, then get rid of the fat before you make gravy with the pan juices. Poach fish instead of frying it, then make a succulent sauce with the poaching water. Steam vegetables, don't boil them; boiling destroys too many vitamins. And when you steam them (using a very small amount of water for best nutritional results), use the water later for a sauce or soup. You will have crisper, tastier vegetables *and* a more nutrient-packed diet.

It's really very easy to become a healthful cook as well as a gourmet cook. All you have to do is get into some new habits.

Look at Your Smoking Habits

If you're a smoker, you probably think I'm going to tell you to stop. Stop worrying; I'm not.

I am going to tell you, in chapter 8, about some of the known effects of cigarette smoking and how it contributes to the degeneration of your body. But no health or self-improvement program can be helpful if it makes your life miserable. You simply won't follow it. You'll find excuses for cheating and, when you do, you'll only be cheating yourself.

You know smoking is not good for you, and by now you're probably sick and tired of hearing just about everyone—including the Surgeon General on every pack of cigarettes you buy—tell you how bad it is. Even the airlines make you sit in the back of the plane.

But if you are so firmly entrenched a smoker that you feel trying to quit would be too rough to be worth it, don't try. The hassle would cause so much stress on your system that you'd just be trading one controllable risk factor for another.

Instead, take comfort from the key word mentioned in chapter 2: *moderation.* You can cut down on your smoking without giving it up altogether—and, if you space out your cigarettes over the day, each one will be more enjoyable, since it will be a special treat instead of a constant habit.

If you are in good general health—that means you're of normal weight and *not* a victim of familial hyperlipidemia—your system can probably tolerate six to ten filtered cigarettes a day without disastrous results. But remember the key word: "moderation." And who knows? If you can cut down to ten a day, maybe you can cut down to seven a day . . . or four . . . or two . . . or six a week . . . or twelve a year . . . or none at all.

Look at Your Blood Pressure

Nowadays you don't have to go to a doctor to find out whether your blood pressure is low, normal or high, although if you go to find out about your blood-lipid level, a blood pressure check will be part of the examination.

High blood pressure is such a dangerous disease—like arteriosclerosis, it usually exists without any symptoms at all until a heart attack or stroke become the tipoff you can't ignore—that public screening programs have been set up all over the country. Some drugstores have blood pressure machines on which you can even "do it yourself." You just insert your arm into a cuff, slip some coins in a slot and the machine does the rest. Charts on the machine will tell you what blood pressure is normal for your age, and whether or not you should see a doctor about the results.

If your blood pressure is high, *please* don't wait to see a doctor for help. Your life could depend on it.

Look at Your Physical Activity

How far do you walk on an average day? Do you park your car as close as possible to your door, then flop into a chair the minute you get through that door? Do you ride buses, subways and taxis for short-distance trips? Do you take the elevator instead of walking up a flight or two? Do you work at a desk from which you seldom get up? Do you prefer watching others play at sports rather than joining in the fun? Do you think joggers, golfers and tennis players are all a little bit crazy? If so, you probably have a waistline to go along with that opinion.

The type of exercise that is best for you will depend upon your age, your weight and the present state of your health. If you have been a slow mover for a long time, a sudden effort to make up for all those lazy years with a strenuous exercise program could be both uncomfortable and very dangerous. Remember the key word "moderation," and see a doctor for a checkup before making any radical change in the amount of exercise you get. This is a serious warning—even more important for people over 40 years of age.

When you have learned what type of exercise is best for you and how much would be helpful instead of harmful, pick an exertion you will enjoy, because the worst enemy of a good exercise program is boredom. Don't strain yourself; entertain yourself with an activity that will be fun as well as fundamentally good for you.

Look at Your Emotional Health

What kind of work do you do? Do you get along well with your family, co-workers and friends? Or are you frequently worn out from arguments and conflicts? Are you lonely, or depressed because no one seems to care?

Such stress factors can contribute to the degeneration of your physical health, as well as promoting a dangerously strong appetite and the feeling that food (especially the rich, sweet, fatty, palate-satisfying kind) is at least a temporary answer to your problems.

There are many answers to the problems of stress, and each person's solution will be different. Some people can find relaxation in enjoyable recreation, which often includes exercise. Others meditate or find help in religion, yoga, biofeedback or even a change of occupation or location. Often, when problems are serious, professional counseling can make a world of difference.

Tension and anxiety are not the only kinds of stress that can harm your physical health. If you feel that your life is boring and too slowly paced, you need something to perk up your spirits, to get you interested in active participation in life, to keep you from pacifying your boredom with fatty foods.

There is a special interest, hobby or enjoyable activity for everyone, no matter what your age, sex, occupation or location. What you need is something to take your mind off whatever is creating stress in your life—and finding it could be the start of a whole new lifestyle, one about which you can be enthusiastic because it will be pointed in the direction of health in every respect.

Stress is endangering your life, your health and your future. Get rid of it by getting involved in something else.

Your Own Preventive Program

Now that you have looked at yourself, your health and your risk factors, you should have a good idea of where to start in putting together your own Personal Prevention Program. I hope this chapter has also given you the urge to get going right away on making the rest of your life a more healthful and enjoyable time.

Most people just need to find out how dangerously they are living in order to make important changes in the right direction. For example, in February of 1981 the ABC-TV program "20/20" broadcast an explanation of coronary risk factors, and asked its viewers to answer a test about them. The producers had expected to get about 40,000 answers—instead they received more than 260,000! The best example of an enthusiastic response was the answer that came in written on the back of an empty candy box; the couple who sent it in wrote: "Because of your test, we threw out the rest."

Throw out the rest of your doubts about what you can personally do to fight the degenerative diseases that lead to arteriosclerosis, heart attack and stroke. It's no longer a matter of debate. In the words of James Schoenberger, M.D., Professor of Preventive Medicine at Rush-Presbyterian-St. Luke's Medical Center in Chicago, "We can't solve the problem with beta or calcium blockers [drugs], heart transplants, coronary bypasses, or other forms of palliative medicine. The only solution is prevention."

Chapter 4

THE INSTITUTE FORMULA: INGREDIENTS 1 THROUGH 9

Can you imagine what would have happened to David if he had faced Goliath without the help of his slingshot? He probably would have been squashed.

The giant you (and all of us) face is Death. While no one can escape him altogether, we now know that we can keep him at a distance for much longer than ever before possible, simply by attacking his advance men: the degenerative diseases that lead to arteriosclerosis, heart attack and stroke. To keep these diseases from squashing us from the inside, we need the same thing David had—not a slingshot, but an effective weapon.

Considering the fact that the pen is generally acknowledged to be mightier than the sword, it's obvious that weapons come in a wide variety of shapes and sizes. Your weapon against premature aging and untimely death is the Institute Program: a combination of low-fat diet, exercise, beneficial lifestyle and now a new, special booster weapon—the Institute Formula.

What is the Institute Formula? A lot of things. It's a food supplement—that is, an addition to the low-fat diet I hope you're already following. It's natural—a mixture of ingredients taken from the earth, the sea and plant life. If you're a victim of familial hyperlipidemia, it's a replacement for the defensive mechanism you lack. If your lipid metabolism is normal, it's an enhancement of your natural defenses.

Technically, the Institute Formula is a compound of what I call the Big Ten: ten specific ingredients that work together to defend your body against the ravages of fatty foods, lethargy and stress. Each of these ingredients alone is good, but put together they're more than just better because each of them contributes something that enhances the effects of the others.

This mutual strengthening is the result of a process scientists call "synergy." Basically, synergy means "working together." To carry the definition a little further, synergy is a system in which two or more individual substances enhance and intensify each other's actions. As a result, the total effect is greater than the sum of its parts.

How does that work? In mathematics, as you know, any time you add specific numbers together, you get a specific total: Three plus three are going to come out six no matter how you arrange them. But in science, when substances work together in synergy, a geometric progression takes place, and each substance becomes stronger—instead of three plus three, you have three *times* three. If you swallowed any one of the Institute Formula's ingredients by itself, the effect would be good. But when you swallow the mixture, the result will not be just better, but *a lot* better—and so will your chances of living a longer, healthier and more energetic life.

Of course, to me the Institute Formula is much more than all that. It is the result of a lifetime, a whole career devoted to search and research, testing and retesting, triumph and discouragement, overcoming discouragement to take the next step in the right direction, finally arriving at the best possible Formula. I hope it will enrich your life half as much as it has mine.

A Little Background Material

What exactly *is* the Institute Formula? The names of the Big Ten ingredients are:

1. Lecithin
2. Phosphatidylcholine
3. Phosphatidyl inositol
4. Phosphatidyl ethanolamine
5. Lethicon
6. Extract of *Chondrus crispus* (Irish moss)
7. Extract of carrageenan
8. Silicon dioxide

9. Niacin
10. Compounded plant extract (mucopolysaccharides)

While you can't quite go out and pick them off a tree and mix them up in your blender, these ingredients are all readily available in nature. And the story of how I (along with a lot of other research physicians, nutritionists and technicians) learned to use them as effective weapons against degenerative diseases and premature aging is a real old-fashioned yarn of drama and discovery, trial and error, success and defeat. Fortunately, the defeats were temporary.

I think it all really began with my own family tree: I have, unfortunately, a very high uncontrollable risk factor in my own heredity, since my father, my mother and all three of her siblings suffered from severe arteriosclerotic diseases.

This is the kind of thing you have to look for in your own family background. One of my mother's brothers died at the age of 52 of coronary heart disease, and before his death had lost his eyesight as a result of the illness. Her other brother died of the cerebral form of atherosclerosis, a cerebral thrombosis (blood clot in the brain). And my mother's sister, the aunt who played an important role in my childhood and helped to bring me up, also suffered from coronary heart failure. As if that weren't enough, many of these relatives' children, my cousins, also died or suffered from atherosclerosis and its complications. My family album was one big picture of uncontrollable risk factor number 4!

Of course, as a child I knew nothing of the implications of my family's health history—and in those days, neither did anyone else. I just knew that my mother was terribly ill and suffering. At the age of 13, when we were living in a small town outside Montreal (where we had moved from London, England, my birthplace), I began taking an active part in my mother's care, taking her to doctors and assisting her with the medications they prescribed. No matter what they did, these learned men could only give my mother a little relief from her suffering; they never were able to cure her. In my frustration over their failure, I decided at that early age to devote my life to medicine and to do my best to discover something new—something that would succeed where the methods and treatments of the early twentieth century had failed.

Becoming a doctor wasn't any easier then than it is now. The numbers were smaller, but it still cost an enormous amount of money to go to college for pre-med training, and medical school. For a while, in an effort to earn enough to pay for my studies, I got sidetracked (I was literally on a side track, since I went to work for the railroads), but destiny has a way of bringing us back to our true direction. It was in working for the railroads that I learned the fascination of research and discovery.

During the years after my initial decision, I read everything I could find about medicine—in a romantic, boyish way—and was profoundly influenced by the book *Arrowsmith*. I was also a very good science student in high school, and won all kinds of prizes. At the same time, I was working very hard to earn the money to put myself through college in the pre-med division.

After graduation from high school, I had to take three years off just to get the money together. Like most youngsters, I took any job I could get my hands on: I was a laborer, a salesman and a postal worker. One day, at age 16, I saw a sign in the post office advertising an open competition for the job of assistant to the chemical engineers in the Canadian government's Forestry Division. Fate, as they say, had struck.

An undue number of accidents had been occurring on the Canadian National Railways because the railroad ties had degenerated from fungus growth. The railroad's chemical engineers had the job of discovering something—some preventive measure—that would protect the ties against the fungus. They needed an assistant, preferably a veteran of World War I who had a Ph.D. degree or at least a Bachelor of Science. I was a 16-year-old with a high-school diploma. But they say it's a lot easier to overcome obstacles if you don't know they're there. In my ignorance of the requirements, I took the examination for the job—and came out first because I had been so good in chemistry!

For three years I worked on the campus at McGill University in Montreal with the chemical engineers, doing work that was a lot more dangerous than I realized at the time. We had to impregnate the railroad ties (and also the telegraph poles that had been infested with the same kind of fungus) with mixtures we hoped would cure the disease. We mixed endless concoctions of creosote in huge cauldrons of boiling oil, trying to determine which mixture would be most effective, most preventive against the fungus infiltration. It was fascinating work; it was *research*.

My duty was to go out on the tracks, dig up the railroad ties and make notes on how much had been eaten by the fungus, before and after the treatments with different creosote mixtures. Finally we hit on one mixture that did the job, and the fungus growth was conquered! The method we discovered is used all over the world now; when you see railroad ties and telegraph poles smeared with a black substance that looks like tar, you will know, "There is Dr. Morrison's first contribution to the prevention of degenerative disease."

That work did a lot more than cure the fungus disease on the railroad ties. It instilled in me a fascination for research that gave specific direction to my already chosen medical career. I wouldn't be just a doctor, I would be a research physician.

The Move to Medicine

After three years I had saved enough money to start pre-med school at McGill University. At the same time it was obvious to me that my mother was getting worse and suffering more. Her deteriorating condition was brought home to me every day—I had to dress her, feed her, comb her hair, help her to walk. After I had been at McGill for a short time, the Canadian climate made her so much worse that we moved to Philadelphia. There she improved, but was still ailing very badly from coronary heart disease, and also arthritis.

In Philadelphia I attended Temple University Medical School and continued to take my mother to the best doctors available. With my medical studies well in progress, I understood a lot more about the methods they were using to try to help her. Synthetic chemicals were being used to relieve her distress. In general the chemicals were satisfactory, but they produced adverse medical reactions called side effects. I knew there had to be something better, but I still had so much to learn.

At Temple, in my sophomore year, I did my first piece of real medical research—and almost didn't live to do the second. I was looking for the causes of degenerative diseases (this time in people, who are a lot more interesting and complicated than railroad ties), and had focused on the liver, an organ that has much to do with metabolism. I organized a team of my fellow students, and we went all over the medical literature, looking for clues, making tests on all kinds of liver diseases.

During the late 20s and early 30s, when I was doing my liver research, no one knew that hepatitis is a virus disease—a highly contagious one. Not having the proper facilities for a controlled research program, we did what a great many medical students and research scientists have done throughout history: We used ourselves as experimental subjects.

In the movies, a scientist who uses himself as a subject usually comes out with two heads, or at least two personalities. In real life, we came out with hepatitis. We were taking blood samples from a ward full of hepatitis patients and using the same needles to take comparative samples from ourselves! We were young, healthy, robust students—but you don't take chances with something as powerful as the hepatitis virus, or with unsterilized needles. Our lesson was learned the hard way—we all became terribly jaundiced and found ourselves on the same ward with our patients, this time as patients ourselves.

I almost died. I spent four months in the hospital with what is called sub-acute atrophy of the liver, a disease in which the liver withers up and loses the power to do its metabolic job. If I had not been so young and basically healthy at that time, I probably would not have lived to continue my research.

But I managed to survive—and in 1932 the results of our research were published in the medical literature. It gives me a great deal of satisfaction to know that this book is being written in the year that marks the fiftieth anniversary of my medical research life.

A Vital Connection

After I graduated from medical school and completed my internship, I continued my research. I was primarily interested in diseases of the liver, since one of them had almost killed me. When I went back to London to study at Guy's Hospital Medical School, I learned that my mother's sister and two brothers were suffering from the same coronary degeneration that had plagued my mother's life. Of course, the pioneering work in the study of heredity had already been done by that time, and many medical students, myself included, had read Charles Darwin's *Origin of Species*, written in 1861. We knew that diseases can be transmitted from one family member to another through genetic patterns, and it was obvious that a pattern for coronary disease ran in my own family.

But Darwin also wrote about other aspects of inheritance. His work indicated that in every organism there is a defense or preservative mechanism operating that protects the host—that is, the human system—from outside attacks by diseases and elements that can lead to disease.

For example, as almost everyone knows now, your body manufactures antibodies to protect you against the bacteria that cause infections. You can still be infected, but when you are, the antibodies rally, strengthen and fight off the infection. In many cases they remain strong enough to keep that particular infection from affecting you again. Once you've had a disease such as measles, your anti-measles antibodies are so strong that you are immune to the disease and can never get it again.

Another example is adrenaline, a substance scientists call "the body's burglar alarm." As pointed out by Hans Selye, M.D., Ph.D., D.Sc., of Montreal (a world-famous expert on stress, and one of the Institute's collaborators), when you are in danger your adrenal glands produce adrenaline to give you a "second wind." The body has had these protectors since the beginning of time, but it remained for us as research physicians to find out about them and develop ways to put them to full use.

It seemed logical to me that the body might also have natural defense substances against the heart disease that ran in my family, but that no one had yet found out about them. The same could be true of the liver, the organ on which I was concentrating my studies at the time. Could there be a connection? I didn't know.

Every research scientist wants to find out everything there is to know, but he has to discipline himself and stick to one subject—and I had committed myself to working on the liver. Little did I know then that my work on the liver was going to lead me into a much broader area, or that the liver and heart were both under attack from a common enemy: saturated fat. If you look up "choline" (the second ingredient of the Institute Formula) in a recent edition of *Dorland's Illustrated Medical Dictionary*, here's what you'll find: "Choline. A vitamin derivable from many animal and some vegetable tissues. It prevents the deposition of fat in the liver." Back in the 30s we didn't know about choline. We did know, however, that fatty deposits in the liver were at least one source of that organ's degenerative diseases.

My work in this area began in earnest in 1935, when I returned from Guy's Hospital Medical School and was assistant gastroenterologist at the Temple University Medical School Hospital. I took care of a number of the wards there, and one of my patients was a 16-year-old boy who was critically ill.

The boy was suffering from continuous infectious disease, the result of a childhood accident. He had not enjoyed a day of good health in many years, and constant illness had weakened him terribly. His liver, in particular, just couldn't stand the strain and became very, very diseased. First he had fatty infiltration, then atrophy (withering) began and soon he was close to death.

I will never forget the day, as I made my rounds in the ward and stopped by his bed, I saw his mother, weeping in despair that her boy was dying. Surely, she pleaded, there was something that medicine could do to save him. Her pleas touched me deeply, and I started giving the case special attention.

After a lot of thought it struck me that, since the boy's liver was diseased, perhaps liver could be used to help him. After all, the ancient Egyptians, five thousand years ago, used a brew made from sheep's livers that was reported to cure liver disease. Hippocrates, known as the Father of Medicine, even mentioned this in his writings.

Egyptian physicians (and priests, who practiced medicine as well as religion in those days) believed that disease in an organ is the result of a breakdown in that organ's natural protective and defensive mechanisms. Therefore, they reasoned, if you provide normal, healthy tissues to replace those that have been broken down by the disease, you can conquer the disease process. I was picking up on an idea that was more than fifty centuries old.

In this century, that idea has been applied in many areas of medicine. For example, extracts from a normal thyroid gland are given to patients who are deficient in it. Insulin, derived from the pancreas, has saved the lives of diabetics who cannot produce the right amounts of insulin on their own. Pituitary extracts are given to patients who lack the pituitary hormone. And the female hormone, estrogen, which comes from the ovaries, is often given to women during and after the menopause to replace the estrogen they lose when their own ovaries stop producing it. The list goes on and on.

The Institute Formula is a result of a branch of this type of therapy—the branch that extracts curative medicinal agents from plants. Originally known as herbal therapy, it is the basis of the pharmaceutical profession on which we rely so heavily today.

One of the first plant derivatives discovered—one that is still widely used—was quinine. It comes from the bark of trees that grow in South America, and has long been known to be effective in the prevention and cure of malaria. Another is digitalis, an extract from the foxglove plant, which is used extensively in the treatment of heart failure and dropsy (an accumulation of fluid in the tissues as a result of heart disease). It was discovered by a nature healer and midwife in England and was reported to be effective in patients by Dr. William Withering as early as 1776.

So, you see, the concept of using organ therapy, as well as plant extracts, to replace deficiencies in organs is well based in centuries of practical application.

In 1935, I applied the replacement concept in a way that must have seemed pretty far out to my young liver patient and his mother. I told the mother that, in 1926, a man named George Minot, M.D., had won the Nobel Prize for having fed great quantities of liver and liver juice to patients who were dying of pernicious anemia. Since her son was terribly anemic (though his anemia was secondary to his disease, not pernicious), I had put two and two together and figured that, if I could build up his liver, antibodies would develop to fight his infection. At the same time, the therapy should help to overcome his anemia.

I instructed the mother to buy all the liver she could find—calves' liver in particular—and pound it into a juice, then have her son drink it. I made special arrangements for her to come into the ward three times a day to feed him.

How dedicated she was—and also very inventive. She spent five or six hours a day going to the slaughterhouses, getting all the livers she could carry, obtaining a bucket of ice from an iceman so they wouldn't spoil, hauling them to her home, and squeezing out the juices by hand—there was, of course, no such thing as an electric blender or food processor in 1935. Then she would mix the liver juice with all kinds of flavors in an effort to make it more palatable for her son. Really, she was inspired!

For the first day or two, the boy vomited the liver mixture right up—it was too much for him, too concentrated, and it assaulted his stomach with a strong dose of the unexpected. So I reduced the dose, and on the smaller amount he began to improve. Then he began to vomit again—the concentration was still too rich. After several months, I realized that he just couldn't take it. The project looked like a failure, but my patient's mother had never given up, even after all she had gone through, and I wasn't about to either.

Finally it occurred to me that, while the liver juice itself was too rich for the boy's system to handle, an extract might be the answer. I contacted our professor of chemistry and some-how persuaded him to help me.

Then it was our turn to haunt the slaughterhouses. We got more fresh livers and packed them in ice, since there were no facilities available for freezing them at the time. I took them to my laboratory and began to make extracts with different chemicals and solvent solutions, falling back on my chemistry background once again. Dr. Robertson helped by making the extracts sterile and free of the impurities that caused reactions.

The boy recovered. It was miraculous! (My word, of course; medical scientists aren't supposed to talk in terms of miracles.) Once the extract was perfected, I began giving him injections as well as small amounts of the liver juices his mother was squeezing out. During all this time, even when the treatment seemed to be failing, she had stubbornly refused to give up, and continued making her daily trips to the slaughterhouses and the iceman, taking the livers home and personally pulverizing them. She saved her son's life. The boy made a wonderful recovery.

Expanding the Idea

I had achieved my first success, using an extract as a weapon against degenerative disease. And I knew the idea couldn't stop there. I also knew that I wasn't the only one working on it; another was Charles Hoagland, M.D., a famous biochemist who was Director of Biochemistry at the Rockefeller Institute (now Rockefeller University) in New York.

When I shared the results of my work with Dr. Hoagland, he offered me a job working with him on perfecting liver extracts at Rockefeller Institute. I wanted to accept, but I couldn't. It was 1937, I was newly married and deeply in debt—I couldn't even pay for my fluoroscope (an instrument used in the office to examine patients). Dr. Hoagland was offering me a salary that wasn't unusual for research scientists in those days, but wasn't enough for my wife, Rita, and me to live on: twenty-five dollars a week. I had to stay at the clinic, working on the wards by day, and moonlighting in my efforts to start my own practice. I borrowed some money, went in with a group of other young doctors and together we started an office practice at night.

Still, I was able to work with Dr. Hoagland, if not *for* him. We developed a liver extract that Lederle Laboratories later manufactured as a product called Intraheptol. It didn't cause a sensation, but it helped a lot of patients with liver diseases.

I published the results of our work in the *Journal of the American Medical Association* (June 21, 1947), and in other medical publications, describing Intraheptol as a supplement to a very low-fat diet, rich in protein and carbohydrates and all the dietary elements that help to build up the body. Other journals published articles about the diet, people began to use it, and Dr. Hoagland and I considered it a small success.

It was a beginning, and a very productive one. I was hopelessly hooked on research by that time, and firmly entrenched in the field of combating degenerative diseases. Meanwhile, the rest of the free world had started combating the Nazi disease. It was 1940 and, like most young men of the time, I entered the military service. As a research physician, I was assigned to work for the Armed Services in Philadelphia as a consultant.

My specialty was gastroenterology, the branch of medicine that deals with the stomach and the rest of the digestive system. So my next idea shouldn't surprise anyone. If extracts of the liver worked so well against certain diseases, why not try extracts of the stomach?

At that time there was no treatment for ulcers except what we called the "Sippy Diet," which consisted mostly of whole milk and rich cream. Of course, whole milk and rich cream are loaded with saturated fats; little did anyone know that while people were curing themselves of ulcers, they were exposing themselves to the dangers of arteriosclerosis.

The Sippy Diet wasn't that effective, either. It helped ease the pain of the ulcer, but didn't do anything to repair the damage in the wall of the stomach.

In the wall of every stomach there is a protective lining called the "gastric mucosa" that protects the stomach from acids and other harsh substances in food. It does its best, but when acids manage to break through the gastric mucosa, the result is an ulcer. I reasoned that extracts of gastric mucosa would strengthen the inner lining of a patient's stomach and help the ulcer to heal.

But where was I going to get extracts of gastric mucosa? I needed animals—lots of them. I also needed a place to work. There was no money to support my research, but from the few dollars I made in private practice, along with some help from Temple University, I managed to squeeze out enough to establish an animal research laboratory.

From animals that had died I made extracts of gastric mucosa. In animals that were still alive I produced experimental ulcers by feeding them an abrasive substance called yellow cincophen. Then I divided them into two groups. Both groups received the same diet of animal feed, but one group (the treatment group) also got my gastric-mucosa extract. The other group (the control group) did not.

The extract cured the ulcers in the treatment group quickly—so fast it was amazing. But the control group, which did not get the extract, did not get cured. So far, so good—in animals. I thought, "I've got to get this to people," but what people? I could not experiment with patients.

I fell back on research scientists' last resort of using relatives as subjects. But this time I didn't use myself, and I certainly knew better than to subject anyone to the dangers my fellow students and I had encountered back in the days of the hepatitis studies. Instead, I asked for volunteers among my students; they were young medical students who understood what they were getting into and were willing to participate in this scientific research. And they knew what to do with the fees I paid them, even though I couldn't afford much.

I paid the student doctors five dollars apiece for their gastric juices—that is, I inserted a tube into each student's stomach and drew out the natural juices that occurred there (no, I didn't give them ulcers). I filtered the gastric juices and neutralized the acid portion to get natural, normal human gastric juices.

I began to feed this natural substance to patients who had peptic ulcers, and shared it with other doctors who did the same; actually, I helped start a Gastric Juice Bank in the U.S. Naval Hospital in Philadelphia. And it worked beautifully! I published my results in the *American Journal of Digestive Diseases* (October 1945).

There was no stopping me after that. If I had ever harbored any doubts that extracts of natural substances could cure degenerative diseases, those doubts had completely disappeared. I felt like a victorious crusader, looking around for a new target to attack.

Back to the Liver—and Beyond

The new target was actually an old one: I went back to working on the liver. That is when I made the dramatic discovery that shaped the rest of my research career and eventually resulted in the creation of the Institute Formula.

In reading the work of Charles Best, M.D., one of the doctors who discovered the value of insulin in treating diabetes, I learned about "lipotropic agents." "Lipo" means "fat," and "tropic" means "a turning." So a lipotropic agent is a substance that can turn fats out of an organ—in other words, get rid of them.

Dr. Best had found that certain lipotropic agents could turn fatty infiltrations out of the livers of experimental animals. I was intrigued; I had to try it for myself. But in order to clear fat out of the liver, you have to have fat there in the first place. How was I going to make my experimental animals fat?

Obesity, you may have noticed, is not a problem with animals, except for some cats and dogs who belong to over-generous people. In nature, animals eat sensibly, and don't get fat. Humans are the only species who eat more than they need to.

So I fed my experimental animals the kinds of diets that make people fat. I used every fatty substance I could get them to swallow—egg yolks, butter, lard and even powdered cholesterol. To their credit, some of them were too smart to eat these foods; I had to force-feed them with tubes.

The diet produced cirrhosis of the liver of the fatty kind very easily, just as it had in Dr. Best's experiments. But then I had an experience with serendipity. "Serendipity" means a valuable and unexpected discovery, such as finding a priceless antique in a junkyard when all you were looking for was a beat-up old vase to hold your flowers. And that's just what happened to me. When the experimental animals died and I performed autopsies on them, I found the fatty degeneration I had expected in their livers, but I also found clumps of fat in their hearts.

I was astonished. I thought, "If this is what I'm finding in the heart, what must there be in the arteries?" It's not hard to guess the answer to that question. The coronary arteries were clogged and blocked with huge lipid deposits. They were literally clogged with fat.

The question then became, How can I prevent that? My work had become a treasure hunt—every discovery provided a clue and an inspiration to go on to the next step. It had also taken on a very personal aspect. After all, I had lost and was continuing to lose members of my own family to coronary heart disease. For them, sadly, my discoveries came too late. But I vowed to devote everything I had to find a way of helping other people escape the same fate.

About this time, another death occurred that reinforced my decision. My wife's mother, in her middle fifties, was critically ill with very advanced coronary arteriosclerosis. She had had a myocardial infarction (heart attack) and a stroke, and had been an invalid for about eight years during what should have been a rich and active period of her life. Although she had been treated by some of the best doctors available, none of them could help her, and she died. With Rita's mother and my mother, the tragedy of arteriosclerosis and heart disease had struck too close to home too often. My interest in the subject was reinforced on an emotional and personal basis, which provided a stimulus even stronger than my professional curiosity and my love of research.

In beginning my work in heart disease, I found I was not alone—or even in on the ground floor—when it came to connecting a fatty diet with degenerative diseases of the circulation. The first work had been done in 1913 by a team of Russian scientists led by Nikolai Anitchkov. Oddly, it seemed to me, no one had paid any attention to his discoveries for thirty years. Even then, when I and a number of others began to pioneer in the field during the post-World War II years, there was controversy. Controversy and, it turned out, a great deal of trouble!

The American Diet Attacked

When I first published reports denouncing the American diet for being too fatty, all hell broke loose. You would have thought I had set fire to the American flag in Yankee Stadium! I had attacked an established all-American institution, and no one was going to let me get away with it.

It is said you must never knock Mom, the flag or apple pie, and you're not in very good shape if you go after baseball and the hot dog, either. I had criticized two out of five, apple pie and hot dogs being among the fatty foods I condemned. Both, in those days, were very heavy in saturated fat: pie crust was made with butter (and the better recipes told you to add lots of butter to the apple mixture as well), while hot dogs in the 30s and 40s were always made of pork, the fattiest meat there is. I'm happy to say that today's pies made with polyunsaturated margarine or vegetable oil taste just as good (you can even buy them frozen if you take the time to read the labels); if you must drastically limit your saturated-fat intake, you can get chicken or turkey hot dogs. (Though you shouldn't eat them too often because of their overall fat content.) But back in the days of Babe Ruth and the Andrews Sisters, I was in trouble.

To me it was obvious that dietary fat intake had a detrimental effect on blood-lipid levels and on the body's vital organs. I had made it happen in experimental animals. I had seen the results with my own eyes when I performed autopsies on the animals and compared them to those who had been fed low-fat diets. And I had read the writings of other investigators who shared my beliefs. Yet for a long time my colleagues and I were outcasts. Today I have to shake my head and sigh as I read an article such as "Diet, Serum Cholesterol, and Death from Coronary Heart Disease" by Richard B. Shekelle, Ph.D., and his colleagues in the Western Electric Study, which appeared in the January 8, 1981 issue of the *New England Journal of Medicine*, one of the most prestigious scientific publications in the world. They wrote:

> *The results [of a twenty-year study of 1,900 men] support the conclusion that lipid composition of the diet affects serum cholesterol concentration and risk of coronary death in middle-aged American men.*

There are many, many more studies that bear out these conclusions, including the work of Ancel Keys, Ph.D., described in chapter 3, and the famous Framingham study directed by my friend, William Kannel, M.D. Recently, 211 researchers from all over the world were sent questionnaires that asked whether they had found and believed that excessive levels of cholesterol in the blood contributed to the development of heart attacks and arteriosclerosis. Based on the results of their own investigations with both animals and human patients, 93 percent of those who responded to the questionnaire answered, "Yes!"

At last we pioneers in the field have been exonerated, at least on the subject of diet. Still, there are some scientists who remain skeptical, and hundreds of thousands of Americans who choose to ignore the facts or think "it only happens to the other guy." These are the people who continue to keep our coronary death statistics in this country way above reasonable limits.

Back in the 40s, however, once I had determined (at least to my own satisfaction) that dietary lipid intake was responsible for a large part of the degeneration that takes place in the body's tissues, the next question was, What can be done about it? The first step was to design a diet that eliminated the major sources of saturated fat. At that time, of course, no one knew about the "good" form of cholesterol (HDL) or even that there was more than one kind; we knew only that high-cholesterol diets blocked the arteries with sticky, gummy globs that slowed the flow of blood. We also knew that the slower blood flows, the more likely it is to clot. And a clot that could easily pass through a normal artery would have a tough time making it through the narrow passages that were blocked by arteriosclerotic plaques. When they couldn't make it through at all, the flow of blood stopped and a heart attack or stroke occurred. It was cholesterol that first created these deadly arterial traffic jams.

How, I wondered, can any of us eat saturated fats such as egg yolks, butter, cream and so on, when these are the very foods we feed to experimental animals in order to create high cholesterol levels? And in every species, we produce coronary heart disease and arteriosclerosis.

To prove the point, I decided to conduct a long-term study of people who already had proven cases of atherosclerosis to see what effects a change of diet would have on their conditions. This study lasted thirteen years. During that time, a great deal more was learned about fats and their effects that helped us to refine our knowledge of degenerative diseases and strike out on many different avenues of cure and prevention. But the original study continued as planned, and the results were no less valid—in fact, the more we learned, the more valid they became.

The diet study group was made up of 100 people who had survived heart attacks and had been discharged from the hospital. I divided them into two groups of 50 and gave one group the low-fat, low-cholesterol diet I had devised. The other 50 were the control group; they kept right on eating the same time-honored (and fat-filled) American diet they had enjoyed all their lives.

It took only three years for the first results to show that I was, indeed, on the right track. Five years later, at the eight-year point, there was no question about it. Of the fifty patients who had kept on eating the fatty American diet, thirty-eight (76 percent) had died of heart attacks or other diseases of the arteries. But in the other group—the fifty people who had followed the low-fat, low-cholesterol diet—only twenty-two (44 percent) had died of the same kinds of illnesses. Considering the possibility of other factors having influenced their life spans, it still remained that almost twice as many patients on low-fat diets had survived as patients on high-fat diets.

Survival wasn't the only factor I measured in this study. It was no surprise that people on the low-fat diet lost weight; it would have been strange if they hadn't. But their weight losses were consistent and brought the added bonus of great improvement in the way they felt. Both men and women lost an average of twenty pounds each, and they lost it slowly, over a period of about three years. No sudden losses, no tired feelings, no hunger pangs—their reducing was safe, gradual and healthful.

And how much better they felt! Let me tell you the story of one patient as an example. She was a typical American housewife with three children whom I'll call Mrs. Rogers (we never use real names in order to protect people's privacy). At the time the diet study began, Mrs. Rogers was 47 years old, had survived a heart attack, and was twenty-five pounds overweight. Before her heart attack she had begun to feel the effects of menopause or "change of life," and was miserable, weak, tired all the time—ready to give up. Her heart attack had seemed like the last straw. Mrs. Rogers made what doctors call a "fairly good" initial recovery from the heart attack. But still she was weak, lethargic and depressed.

After a year on the low-fat diet, she was a different woman. Not only had she lost twenty-five pounds, but everyone noticed that the woman who had been hiding under all that excess tonnage was attractive, vivacious and bright, with a zest for living that was intensified by her knowledge that she had come close to death. Her family could hardly believe the transformation that had taken place; her home was once again a cheerful place to be.

Not the least of the beneficiaries of the change was her husband, who confided to me that his wife's former depression had been contagious—and he had caught it. Her new cheerfulness and enthusiasm also proved to be catching, and Mr. Rogers began looking forward to coming home in the evening rather than dreading it. It was, he told me, like rediscovering his wife as she had been in her youth.

If that story sounds like a commercial for a product, I guess it is, but the product is good health and nutrition rather than something you can buy. It was far from an isolated occurrence—others in the low-fat diet group also found that as they lost weight they gained strength, vitality and good spirits, and once again were able to work and take part in leisure activities they thought they had lost with their youth.

More Than a Diet

As I mentioned, the diet study took thirteen years, but a lot more than the role of diet was learned about fats and degenerative diseases during that time. For one thing, the part played by heredity was explored.

In a group of 200 patients who had heart attacks, my colleagues and I discovered that a great many seemed to be links in chains of heredity—that is, they belonged to families in which heart disease was a common occurrence. We reasoned that some kind of special susceptibility ran in these families, but we didn't yet know what it was.

Later, David Adlersberg, M.D., and Charles Wilkinson, Jr., M.D., learned that some people did, indeed, inherit an inability to metabolize fats, and that these were the same people who tended to have heart attacks and other diseases of the circulation. Often it was possible, just by studying a family history, to accurately predict whether or not a given person was likely to have angina (chest pain), high blood pressure or a heart attack.

Genetic laws are not precise for individuals, but they come pretty close. Hereditary tendencies, as I've mentioned before, skip some members of families and land on others, and there's no way of telling *exactly* which individuals will or will not be affected. But if you are a member of a heavily heart-attack-stricken family, the odds are definitely against you, whereas if few or no members of your family have been afflicted by degenerative diseases leading to heart attacks, your chances of escaping them are much better.

Good research scientists are always open to the suggestion that something they haven't even thought of may be affecting the outcome of their studies. So they search for other possibilities in addition to evaluating what they think is causing a disease. In the case of the many heart-disease studies that took place in the post-war years, cholesterol was only one of the many possible villains being investigated.

In our study of the 200 patients in whom we found strong hereditary traits for heart disease, my colleagues and I discovered that the great majority had excesses of fats in their blood. But we also found patients with normal cholesterol levels. What had caused *their* heart attacks?

Some were the victims of other fat abnormalities—and so we learned that cholesterol was not working alone in the heart-attack business. Four other fat components were also labeled "public enemies" by early investigators: beta lipoproteins (now known as LDL), fat enzymes that worked as activators of cholesterol, chylomicrons (see chapter 2) and special large complexes of fat molecules that were discovered by John Gofman, Ph.D., and a team of biophysicists.

So we were up against a multitude of factors, not just one. We had learned that it is possible for a person to have a perfectly normal cholesterol level and still be at high risk of heart attack because of abnormalities in the metabolism of any of the other fat components. Still, cholesterol appeared to be the most important factor, and when it could be lowered or controlled at least one battle in the war against heart disease was being won.

It followed that, if there was more than one fat abnormality at the root of the problem, there must be more than one method of attack. The low-fat, low-cholesterol diet produced very promising results, but it was still in its experimental stages and being followed by very few people. Was there a way, we wondered, of preventing the absorption of fats in people who continued to eat dangerously fatty foods?

Probably no one knows exactly how many substances, mixtures, drugs, food supplements and other concoctions were tested, but the number must have been enormous. Most failed and were discarded, but some succeeded—and a few succeeded so well that they found their way into the present Institute Formula.

To tell you their story, I'm going to go down the list of Formula ingredients one by one. By the time I'm through, you'll understand just how unique this new food supplement is, how it works, and what it can do for you.

Ingredient Number 1: Lecithin

First of all, what is it? The word "lecithin" comes from the Greek *lethikos*, which means "yolk of egg"—and that terminology can cause a lot of confusion right off the bat. If lecithin comes from egg yolks, which are known to be one of the heaviest sources of cholesterol, how can it help to eliminate cholesterol from the blood?

The answer is that there are several types of lecithin. And this fact *is* confusing. When lecithin was first publicized as a weapon against cholesterol, manufacturers rushed to produce it in commercial form, and people rushed to health food stores to buy it in capsule, tablet and granular form. But not everyone knew that you have to be very careful of the *type* of lecithin you're taking. You have to consider the source.

Surprisingly, some research physicians do not even make the necessary distinction. As late as 1979, twenty-one years after the publication of my first study on the lipid-lowering power of lecithin, my old friend David Kritchevsky, Ph.D., and his colleagues at the Wistar Institute of the University of Pennsylvania in Philadelphia published a report on a study of rabbits fed a low-cholesterol diet augmented with saturated fatty lecithin. After six months of this combination, the doctors found that the rabbits had not lost any weight and had higher cholesterol levels and higher ratios of LDL to HDL than did ordinary rabbits.

Of course the rabbits had high levels of cholesterol and LDL—the lecithin used in the study was egg-yolk lecithin. And the so-called "low-cholesterol" diet was 14 percent hydrogenated coconut oil. These are the two heaviest sources of saturated fat on record.

According to this group of researchers, their "results suggest that phosphatides [lecithin] do not affect the course of atherosclerosis in rabbits"; they conclude that "lecithin has no effect upon atherosclerosis." The conlcusion I draw from these statements is that anyone who cares for his health should be as careful in choosing lecithin as he is in picking mushrooms in the woods.

Lecithin exists in almost every living tissue. It is an essential constituent of animal and vegetable cells. But please remember, there are several varieties of lecithin; some contain saturated fatty acids (those that come from egg yolks, for example), while others provide unsaturated fatty acids.

The lecithins that contain saturated fatty acids can be hazardous to your health. This was pointed out to the public in the magazine *Science* in a 1979 article by Norman L. Gershfeld, Ph.D., of the National Institute of Arthritis, Metabolism, and Digestive Diseases. Calling these lecithins "disaturated," Dr. Gershfeld wrote:

> *If they adsorb [stick] to arterial walls as they do to glass and polystyrene surfaces, there may be increased probability of atherosclerosis when the disaturated lecithin content of plasma is elevated . . . a high concentration of disaturated lecithin in plasma may be a significant risk factor for atherosclerosis, independent of triglyceride and cholesterol concentrations.*

So be careful! The lecithin that is used in the Institute Formula—and the kind you should be sure to get if you buy lecithin as a food supplement—is polyunsaturated *soya lecithin*, extracted from soybeans.

Why not just eat soybeans? For the same reason I fed liver extracts to my 16-year-old patient back in 1935. If you ate as many soybeans as it would take to give you the amount of soya lecithin contained in the Institute Formula, they would make you sick—just as huge amounts of liver were rejected by my patient's system. Extraction takes the important elements from a natural source and discards the rest, so you get, so to speak, your cake without having to eat it, too.

Take a multivitamin tablet, for example. An ordinary multivitamin tablet is just a little bigger than an aspirin; it's pretty easy to swallow. Now look at the label on the bottle it came in. There is a long list of ingredients, and you're getting so many milligrams of each one. It takes a lot more space to cram all that information on the label than it does to squeeze the vitamin extracts into a tiny tablet. That's the beauty of extracts. We eliminate the middleman and give you the goods, right up front—it's "no-frills" nutrition, pure and simple.

Why not just take pills? Because eating is too much fun. Besides, foods contain other essentials that tablets can't provide—fiber, for example. I doubt the day will ever come when people live exclusively on extracts, as some science-fiction movies have predicted. The best of both worlds is to eat the foods that are good for you and provide so much enjoyment, then take supplements such as the Institute Formula for all the necessary extracts, like lecithin.

What, exactly, is lecithin? Technically, it's a "phosphatide," which means it contains the natural element phosphorus. In the early days of my research, when my colleagues and I were searching for substances to use in fighting heart disease, we went through hundreds and hundreds of compounds, in tissue cultures, organ cultures and experimental animals, until we found two categories that worked: the mucopolysaccharides and the phosphatides (more about the mucopolysaccharides later). And lecithin and its derivatives turned out to be the most effective.

Lecithin is also a phospho*lipid*, meaning it is a *fat* that contains phosphorus. As mentioned earlier, some lecithins contain saturated fats, while others contain unsaturated fats. We are going to ignore the saturated ones, which should be avoided, and concentrate on the good lecithin, *soya lecithin.*

Lecithin includes mainly phosphatidylcholine and phosphatidyl ethanolamine—but, as you may have noticed, those are the names of Ingredients Number 2 and Number 4 in the Institute Formula. Confusion can reign if we don't get these two ingredients straightened out right at the beginning. Lecithin (Ingredient Number 1) is made up of phosphatidylcholine (Ingredient Number 2) plus phosphatidyl inositol (Ingredient Number 3), plus phosphatidyl ethanolamine (Ingredient Number 4). Why are they considered four different ingredients? Because each is a different concentration, a different extraction. Lecithin is the natural compound of all of them, and each of the others, when used as an ingredient of the Formula, is a stronger concentration than that found in natural lecithin. That's one reason why the total effect of the Institute Formula is greater than the sum of its parts.

Soya lecithin is a phospholipid containing polyunsaturated fats. As you know from chapter 2, polyunsaturated fats are necessary to health, and you have to get them from your diet because the body does not manufacture them. Soybeans and soybean oil are excellent sources of lecithin, but to get the real benefit of this essential phospholipid, informed people have been adding it to their diets in the form of supplements, the best being soya lecithin granules. Now, with the Institute Formula, you can have this benefit as well as the help of all the other ingredients mixed together.

If you are a label reader in the supermarket, you may have noticed that lecithin is listed as an ingredient in a number of products (biscuits, crackers and margarine, for example). As you know, oil and water don't mix—yet both are present in our bodies as well as in commercially prepared foods. Emulsifiers, such as lecithin, have the ability to hold oil molecules and water molecules together—in fact, when I first started working with lecithin, it was being used widely in industry to hold chemical products together. But the amounts of lecithin found in packaged foods are so small (usually no more than 0.1 or 0.2 percent) that they won't do you much good nutritionally. You still need the Institute Formula.

A New Use for Lecithin

I discovered the anti-degenerative value of lecithin almost by accident. Once I had been convinced that blood-lipid levels strongly influenced the presence or absence of degenerative diseases (especially those that led to arteriosclerosis, heart attack and stroke), I began studying the lipid levels of patients to whom I had access in the hospitals in which I worked. Among these patients were a number of people who were being given soybeans and soybean protein for nutrition because they had lactose intolerance—that is, the inability to tolerate milk. It didn't take me long to notice that the levels of total lipids (particularly cholesterol) in the lactose-intolerant people became lower on the soybean diet. (In those days, no one knew about the different types of cholesterol—the good guys and bad guys, or HDL and LDL-VLDL—so we concentrated on total lipids and total cholesterol.) There were lots of other factors that had to be considered—for one thing, these people were *not* getting the saturated fats they would have received if they had been able to stand milk; nevertheless, the levels of total lipids fell, and did so pretty quickly when the soybean-extract programs were begun.

That's how I became interested in lecithin. I wasn't the only one interested in lecithin, however, and I wasn't even the first one to publish an article on the subject. In 1943, while I was getting started and putting my two and two together, Dr. David Adlersberg and Harry Sobotka, Ph.D., of New York's Mount Sinai Hospital published the results of a preliminary study in that hospital's journal. The opening lines of their article clearly show what an early stage we were at then, even in defining the role of cholesterol in heart disease. They wrote:

> *The significance of hypercholesterolemia [too much cholesterol] is not well established. It may lead in some instances to severe organic changes, particularly in the cardiovascular apparatus.*

But they had recognized the lipotropic (lipid-lowering) effects of lecithin, and were able to give 10 to 70 grams of soya lecithin daily to five patients in the form of cookies. When their study began, all five patients had very high cholesterol levels, ranging from 360 milligrams to an extreme of 1,420 milligrams (remember, the normal range is between 150 and 250 milligrams).

The cholesterol levels of all the patients went down as long as they ate their lecithin-laced cookies every day (three patients took 15 grams per day; the other two got 12 grams per day). But when they stopped, their cholesterol levels started to go back up. Drs. Adlersberg and Sobotka summarized their study by stating:

> *Five cases of xanthomatosis [fatty lumps, chapter 2] and hypercholesterolemia showed a striking decrease of the serum cholesterol level upon prolonged feeding of lecithin. A few months after the feeding of lecithin was interrupted, the serum cholesterol returned to the original high figures. Further therapeutic trials are suggested.*

"Further therapeutic trials are suggested"—that was all I needed to hear to stimulate my own interest.

I conducted my "trial" a little bit differently, though. The compound that Drs. Adlersberg and Sobotka had given their patients in cookies was 20 percent lecithin and 30 percent soybean oil (the remaining 50 percent, other ingredients). The oil, I thought, contributed an unknown factor, and I wanted to find out what effect the lecithin alone would have. So I used 36 grams of lecithin per day in my study (more than twice the amount the other doctors had used).

I also knew that other studies had succeeded in lowering cholesterol levels 15 to 20 percent with lecithin, without dietary restrictions. But I was thinking big. I wanted to lower the levels *more* than 25 percent—and use my low-fat diet as well as lecithin.

To make the test really tough (we call that "critical standards of evaluation" in the literature), I chose twenty-one hypercholesterolemic patients who had already been through other efforts at lowering their cholesterol levels—without success. They weren't strangers, or names pulled out of a hat—all of them had been my patients for at least ten years, and all of them had been following a 25-grams-of-fat-per-day diet I had prescribed. Every one had a cholesterol level of above 300 milligrams.

I quickly learned that some people can't take large doses of lecithin. Six of my patients had bad reactions, including stomach pains, skin rashes and nausea. In those cases I stopped giving lecithin, or reduced the dosage to an amount they could tolerate. All six had to be taken out of the study.

I was left with fifteen patients, four men and eleven women, ranging in age from 38 to 80 years—one was a 52-year-old woman whose cholesterol level at the start of the study was a frightening 1,012 milligrams! I took blood samples from them once a month, and analyzed the samples to see what was happening to their cholesterol levels.

At the end of three months, twelve of the fifteen patients had experienced striking reductions in cholesterol levels (the average was 41 percent). The other three had problems that could have affected the results: One was taking a steroid hormone for rheumatoid arthritis, the second had to take medicine that interfered with food absorption, and the third had emotional problems and wouldn't stick to the low-fat diet. But those who stuck to the diet and took the lecithin could only be called successes.

Most remarkable (and certainly most gratifying to me) was the woman who had started the study with a cholesterol level of 1,012 milligrams. At the end of three months, her level was down to 186 milligrams—within normal limits! I couldn't have been happier—and neither could she.

I reported the results of this study in the medical journal *Geriatrics* in January of 1958. By that time a lot of other researchers had jumped on the lipid-lowering bandwagon, and a wide variety of agents had been tested and reported. But I was able to confidently state in the summary of my article: "Lecithin was found to be the most effective cholesterol-lowering agent tested to date." Of course, I meant soya lecithin.

Lipoproteins Identified

After that study (which has since been referred to as a "classic" by a number of other researchers), I went on to other fields, conducting studies on choline and mucopolysaccharides. But other investigators continued to work with lecithin, and many, many reports were published, some of which I'll describe.

Meanwhile, much more was being learned about the mechanism of arteriosclerosis and the nature of lipid metabolism. Perhaps the most significant breakthrough was the identification of HDL cholesterol (which works *against* arteriosclerotic plaque formation) and LDL and VLDL cholesterols (which *promote* arteriosclerotic plaque formation). No longer could we simply measure cholesterol levels; now we had to break the cholesterol down and find out what *kinds* people had, and in what amounts. The battle was getting much more complicated.

Today we still don't know all the answers, but the amount we've learned is incredible! In 1979, the current concepts about the way HDL works were summarized by John A. Glomset, M.D., of the University of Washington in Seattle, who reported that HDL may:

1. remove cholesterol from cells;
2. remove cholesterol from the surface remnants of triglyceride-rich lipoproteins; or
3. be involved in the transport of polyunsaturated fatty acids.

In 1980, an entire issue of the important journal *Circulation*, published by the American Heart Association, was devoted to an extensive study of HDL called the "Lipid Research Clinics Program Prevalence Study," led by H. A. Tyroler, M.D., of the University of North Carolina. The study was undertaken, Dr. Tyroler explained in his introduction, because:

> *interest in HDL cholesterol, relatively dormant since the 1950s, was heightened by the rediscovery in the 1970s of the negative association of HDL cholesterol with coronary heart disease within a wide range of geographic, ethnic, social, age, sex, and race groups. The magnitude of the association has been found to be as large or larger than that of the major known risk factors.*

That doesn't mean you should ignore the risk factors—not by a long shot. But it does mean that the discovery of lecithin's power to *increase* your level of HDL has taken on a much greater significance.

The 70s were a boom decade for lipid research, and lecithin had its share of research studies and published reports—so many that even to list them all, much less describe them, would tax your patience. However, I've selected some as an example of what we have learned, just to bring home how important soya lecithin is to you, and why it is an important ingredient in the Institute Formula.

1974—New Avenues

In order to determine "potential new avenues of investigation that may prove fruitful in conjunction with programs already underway or in the planning stages," Carlos Krumdieck, M.D., Ph.D., and C. E. Butterworth, Jr., M.D., of the University of Alabama undertook a review of atherosclerosis based on the following general concepts:

> *a) atherosclerosis, at least prior to the development of scarring, fibrosis, and calcification, must be a reversible disorder;*
> *b) it should not be considered an inescapable consequence of aging; and*
> *c) it should be understood as a syndrome, the pathogenesis [development] of which is associated with both elevation of circulating lipids and a variety of factors resulting in vascular injury.*

I couldn't help having a feeling of *déjà vu* when I read that—it sounded like a replay of the opening of my 1948 paper in the *American Journal of Medical Science:*

Arteriosclerosis and other diseases of premature aging
are disorders of lipid metabolism and not the result of
"wear and tear" of the arteries as is commonly assumed.

Your past deeds do come back to haunt you—but in this case, I'm glad. There was a fatalism and sense of inevitability associated with premature aging and arteriosclerosis back then, a belief that nothing could be done to stay the hand of the Grim Reaper with his scythe of death. I challenged that concept then, and now, more than thirty years later, it is universally accepted.

Drs. Krumdieck and Butterworth were reporting on their survey of the effectiveness of both soya lecithin and vitamin C in controlling the development of atherosclerosis. (Although I heartily endorse the use of vitamin C, the subject at hand is lecithin, so I'll stick to what they said about that.) Their findings add emphasis to my warnings about being careful to choose the right kind of lecithin, since they compared medical research on both the saturated (egg yolk) and polyunsaturated (soybean) forms and concluded

> *not all lecithins will serve equally well . . . only those*
> *lecithins bearing polyunsaturated fatty acids . . . would*
> *favor the removal of cholesterol deposits. Saturated lec-*
> *ithins would not do this.*

They credited another group of researchers for finding that

> *the administration of polyunsaturated lecithin derived*
> *from soybean not only accelerated the resorption of cho-*
> *lesterol much more effectively than the relatively satu-*
> *rated lecithins from eggs, but in effect prevented the*
> *development of cholesterol induced atheroma [plaques]*
> *in the rabbit.*

Soybean Lecithin Makes the News

That same year, 1974, an anonymous newswriter brought the point home in an article in *Medical World News* (a magazine that is to doctors what *Time* and *Newsweek* are to everyone else). The author wrote:

> *Diets high in polyunsaturates have long been considered*
> *standard preventive measures to be taken in cases of*
> *arteriosclerosis-prone patients with high cholesterol lev-*

els. Now soybean lecithin, with its super-high polyun-
saturated fatty acid content, seems to hold out hope for
really effective treatment of the disease. While lecithin
from animal sources contains only about 40 percent of
polyunsaturates, soybean has from 65 percent to 75
percent.

The article reported on the work of Dr. Hubert H. Peeters and a team of doctors at the Simon Stevin Research Institute in Bruges, Belgium, who had tried giving soybean lecithin to Type II hyperlipidemic patients by injecting it intravenously. After fourteen days, "the patients experienced a marked lowering of lipids in the bloodstream," they reported, "especially excess plasma cholesterol, which was diminished by 40 percent." Soybean lecithin had also significantly lowered their levels of LDL, which is, according to the European doctors, "now accepted as the real cause of Type II arteriosclerosis."

Dr. Peeters commented that polyunsaturated lecithin is "a nontoxic, natural product with no local reaction and no side effects observed in the organs. It can be in the stomach for a long time and present no problems, regardless of age and sex."

In 1976, Mark Bricklin, executive editor of the popular health magazine *Prevention,* wrote an article in which he described the 1943 work of Drs. Adlersberg and Sobotka, as well as my own study published in 1958. In that story he dubbed lecithin a "cholesterol cop," a nickname I liked very much. As a cop, lecithin has a pretty impressive arrest record.

Lecithin "Down Under"

Early in 1975, in Sydney, Australia, L. A. Simons, M.D., was trying his best to lower lipid levels in a family that suffered from hereditary hyperlipidemia on a grand scale. He tried diets; he tried drugs. Nothing worked. Suddenly, and without any change in diets or drug therapy, several of the family's members showed dramatic drops in blood cholesterol levels, and marked improvements in their conditions.

Baffled, Dr. Simons questioned his patients closely and found that, in each case, the person had begun taking lecithin on his own before the plunge in cholesterol level. No doctor is ever going to recommend self-medication to a patient, but in some cases, serendipity occurs. These patients had stumbled onto an answer that their doctor had completely overlooked.

Dr. Simons was intrigued, and determined to find out for himself whether the lecithin had done the trick, or whether the cholesterol-level drops could perhaps be attributed to something else that "ran in the family." He began a test with ten people, none of whom were related to one another.

Three of these people were hospital employees with normal cholesterol levels; seven were patients with hyperlipidemia. Four (including the three employees) were told to continue eating their regular diets; the other six were kept on the low-cholesterol diets they had been following for several months.

Dr. Simons started out giving these patients 13½ grams of soya lecithin each day, then increased the dose to between 20 and 30 grams a day. Some were also given a drug called clofibrate, known to lower plasma lipid levels.

"Lecithin alone produced significant reductions in plasma cholesterol concentration in one out of three normal subjects, and in three out of seven patients with hypercholesterolemia," Dr. Simons reported in the *Australian and New Zealand Journal of Medicine* in 1977. He also noted that one patient, who was taking clofibrate alone, added safflower oil to his diet for two weeks. The oil contained the same amount of linoleic acid as did 30 grams of soya lecithin—and the man's cholesterol level fell accordingly after he began using the oil.

Why is linoleic acid important? "Depending on its source, lecithin may contain a high proportion of linoleic acid," Dr. Simons wrote, pointing out that soya lecithin is the proper source. "Diets rich in linoleic acid are well capable of suppressing plasma cholesterol concentrations," he continued, "and this observation may justify the clinical use of lecithin."

He made another very important point: "Most of the change in plasma cholesterol concentration, when it occurred, was due to a reduction in beta lipoproteins [LDL]." Almost as a bonus, the Australian doctor commented that "lecithin was well tolerated by all subjects without adverse side effects."

A Challenge Met

Whenever anything becomes as popular as lecithin was getting to be in the 1970s, you can be certain someone is bound to find fault with it. This has happened to lecithin—to this day there are doctors who refuse to accept the results of widespread lecithin research—but no one has yet offered a challenge that can't be met with facts. Let me give you an example.

In August of 1978, the *New York State Journal of Medicine* published a question from an unidentified reader, "Is lecithin effective in the prophylaxis [prevention] and treatment of hyperlipidemia?"

The writer who answered the question (he or she was not identified either) cited a 1974 study by H. F. ter Welle, M.D., in which soya lecithin had been given to twelve hyperlipidemic patients for about five months. At the end of that time, Dr. ter Welle had "concluded that there was no significant influence on the lipid parameters under investigation."

After describing another failure in which twenty-five patients had taken lecithin plus cynarine (an ingredient of artichoke) without notable results, the respondent stated, "There is no evidence that lecithin . . . is effective in lowering serum cholesterol and preventing heart disease."

Sounds discouraging, doesn't it? But wait, there's a catch. Dr. ter Welle had given his subjects 1.2 grams of lecithin per day; the other study's patients had received 550 milligrams (a little more than half a gram) per day. When I conducted my first study in 1958, I gave patients up to *36 grams per day!* A check of other research projects confirms the fact that a little lecithin is not enough. A pinch of pepper won't liven up your stew, and a dab of lecithin won't lower your lipid level. These investigators had simply not used enough lecithin to get favorable results!

There is no hard-and-fast rule as to how much lecithin a person has to take per day. Remember, some people have normal cholesterol levels, and others have dangerously high cholesterol levels. Some people have familial hyperlipidemia, and others don't. In general (*very* general), the average preventive amount is about 4 grams per day for normal people. Those who have had a heart attack or stroke and are trying to rebuild their health will probably need about 10 grams a day. But please notice that I'm hedging and being vague, using words such as "average" and "about." Each person is different, and each person's needs are different. Recommended dosages will be discussed when I tell you how to use the Institute Formula in chapter 5.

An Established Fact

The reports go on and on. From Italy in 1978:

> *Soybean polyunsaturated phosphatidylcholine [lecithin]*
> *was given orally to 21 hyperlipidemic patients for 120*
> *days. A significant reduction was found in serum total*

lipids, cholesterol, triglycerides, pre-beta [VLDL], and beta [LDL] lipoproteins. No adverse side effect was observed.
—Current Therapeutic Research

From England and West Germany in 1979:

Polyunsaturated lecithin may modify the atherogenic process . . . this would underline the necessity of maintaining a sufficient plasma concentration of polyunsaturated lecithin.
—Medizinische Welt

From Rutgers University, New Jersey, in 1980:

The biochemical data indicate that oral polyunsaturated lecithin can modify plasma lipoprotein concentration. It is suggested that dietary polyunsaturated lecithin may alter lipoprotein composition to exert a favorable effect on lipoprotein transport in patients with hyperlipidemia, supporting the anti-atherogenic effect reported by others.
—American Journal of Clinical Nutrition

And from Los Angeles in 1980: Four men and one woman, aged 64 to 84 years, followed a low-fat diet and took 10 grams of soya lecithin per day for two years.

The average reduction of 22 percent in serum cholesterol and 26 percent in triglycerides . . . was achieved by a diet low in fat and cholesterol, supplemented with lecithin. The results are important because all of the participants were able to follow the diet protocol while continuing their normal activities, and did so willingly and eagerly over the entire 26-month period.
—American Journal of Surgery

Interviewed by writer Tom Voss of *Prevention* about the Los Angeles study, Ronald Tompkins, M.D., of the UCLA School of Medicine stated, "At this point we're not certain, but we think that it may be important to combine lecithin with a low-fat diet to really do the trick."

I agree heartily. I also believe that it's important to combine lecithin with the other ingredients in the Institute Formula as well as with exercise and regulation of stress. That's what the Institute Program is all about.

Ingredient Number 2: Phosphatidylcholine

Rather than be ponderous (there seems to be an unwritten rule that scientific language has to be ponderous), I'm going to call this ingredient simply "choline" without the "phosphatidyl."

All "phosphatidyl" means is that choline is a phosphatide; it is the main component of lecithin. But, as Ingredient Number 2 of the Institute Formula, it is a special concentration, a stronger form than the choline you get automatically when you take lecithin.

The percentage of choline in the lecithin we use—that is the natural derivative from the soybean state—is about 25 to 35 percent. But when we purify and extract further, we can double or triple the potency of the choline. This increases synergy and strengthens the effect of the improvement choline makes in lipid metabolism.

Choline is a member of the vitamin B complex. It contains an enzyme (activator) called "lecithin-cholesterol acyltransferase" (LCAT) that plays a very important part in breaking up dangerous cholesterol so that it can be transported out of the system instead of sticking to the walls of the arteries. Choline acts as an energizer that helps to set this cleansing process in motion.

Choline also prevents the deposition of fat in the liver, as I mentioned earlier in this chapter. A form of choline has been used to correct diseases such as fatty degeneration and cirrhosis of the liver.

But that's not all. A more recent discovery is that choline acts as a neurotransmitter—that is, a substance that aids in the transmission of nerve impulses throughout the body from the brain. Why is this important to the study of degenerative diseases that lead to arteriosclerosis, heart attack and stroke? Because it has been shown that mental and emotional stress contribute to these diseases, partly by interfering with choline as it tries to do its job as a neurotransmitter.

What is choline's job as a neurotransmitter? Let's look at it step by step, again using a method of transportation as an example.

As a neurotransmitter (called acetylcholine), choline is somewhat like the third rail that makes it possible for a subway or electric commuter train to move from station to station. Without the electricity in the third rail, these vehicles couldn't move.

And without choline, necessary nerve impulses could not travel from one nerve cell to another.

The normal travel of these nerve impulses is responsible for our ability to move with what we call "coordination," and even to think and remember. Without normal movement of the nerve impulses, we would become physically awkward and mentally forgetful. In a study of thirty male volunteers (reported in 1979 by a team of researchers in Baltimore), administration of choline, both with and without lecithin, was shown to improve memory by 30 percent over a three- to four-month period.

Another example of the way neurotransmitters work is the "funny bone." At one time or another you have probably bumped your elbow in that certain spot between the bones and felt a temporary sensation that's a lot like an electric shock running down your arm. A momentary paralysis occurred, with electriclike tingling, and even numbness in your hand. You probably didn't like the reaction much, but it didn't last long and left no ill effects, so you just forgot about it.

But a lot was going on in the minute or two that the "funny-bone" feeling lasted. First of all, you struck the nerve in your elbow, a very sensitive nerve that doesn't take well to being hit. It reacted by "screaming" in its own unique way—by sending (through the enzyme activated by choline) a lightninglike transmission to all the nerve cells along its pathway. Without choline, the enzyme would not be activated, and the transmission of the feeling would not occur. However, the transmission of other, essential nerve impulses also would not occur, and you'd be in big trouble.

Still, what does all this have to do with cholesterol and plaques sticking to the arteries? Just this: Nervous stress causes exhaustion of the choline-activated neurotransmitters—and that exhaustion has been shown to increase the levels of harmful cholesterol in the blood.

Therefore:

Step 1. Choline activates the movement of essential nerve impulses along their pathways—as electricity activates the movement of an electric train along its track.

Step 2. Mental and emotional stress exhaust the neurotransmitters, slowing down the movement of the nerve impulses—as a brownout slows the movement of trains along the electric track.

Step 3. The slowdown of nerve impulses contributes to a rise in cholesterol level—as a slowdown of trains contributes to a rise in the number of commuters angrily waiting for their transportation.

Step 4. Choline from outside the body (as in the Institute Formula) is added to the system to pep up the exhausted neurotransmitters—as the restoration of full electric power gets the trains moving back on schedule.

Step 5. The cholesterol level goes back to normal (or wherever it was before the choline "brownout")—as the commuter congestion is relieved by a return to normal traffic movement.

These conclusions were reached after many studies into the effects of stress on cholesterol levels. For example, the Western Association of Research has shown that accountants going through the stress of income tax time have elevated blood cholesterol levels. And John Peterson, M.D., Professor of Medicine at Loma Linda University in California, has shown the same to be true of medical students when they're under the stress of final examinations.

Coincidence? No. In these research studies it was found that cholesterol measurements returned to their previous levels, or to normal levels, after the periods of emotional and mental stress were over. Nervous exhaustion therefore causes cholesterol levels to rise; choline can help to correct the exhaustion, thus lowering the cholesterol levels.

My Research into Choline

During my earlier work, I had discovered that choline is the main component of lecithin. After my experiments with lecithin, I began to use choline in its pure form, and worked with chemists to prepare different forms and concentrations. Eventually I arrived at the one we use now, phosphatidylcholine (also called EPL, which stands for "essential phospholipids"). My reasoning was that, since choline is the main constituent of lecithin, it was important to investigate them both.

I published the results of my choline investigation in the July, 1949, issue of *Geriatrics*. The study started in 1946, after it had been established that high lipid levels had a lot to do with atherosclerosis and the speed with which it developed. My first studies showed that choline could affect the way atherosclerosis developed in animals.

I gave choline, along with cholesterol, to groups of laboratory rabbits, with truly convincing results. When the rabbits got a small amount (0.5 milligrams) of choline, the substance prevented atherosclerosis in 55 percent of them. When the dosage was increased to 1 gram a day, the choline prevented atherosclerosis in 78 percent. Choline had saved a lot of rabbits!

Now it was time to adapt these good results to helping people. I wanted to use people who already had arteriosclerotic heart disease, to see what effect choline might have on their chances of living longer. I was able to assemble from the wards of the 4,100-bed Los Angeles County General Hospital a group of 230 patients who had suffered heart attacks, had been treated and had been released from the hospital.

My colleague, William F. Gonzalez, M.D., and I divided the 230 patients into two equal groups—115 would get choline in addition to their regular post-heart-attack treatment, and the other 115 would have the regular treatment alone.

The groups were about as much alike as we could make things. For example, there were seventeen women and ninety-eight men in the group that would get choline (the treated group), and twenty-one women and ninety-four men in the other group (the control group). The patients in the treated group were between 28 and 70 years old, while those in the control group were between 30 and 70.

Our studies with animals had shown Dr. Gonzalez and me that we got the best results when we gave the animals as much choline as they could take. So we started out by giving the treated group 32 grams a day of choline. But like the liver juices administered to my 16-year-old patient, that turned out to be too much. Some of the patients couldn't take it—they had very painful stomachaches caused by inflammation of the stomach's lining. So we reduced the dosage until we settled on 12 grams a day, which they took by mouth.

After they left the hospital, all 230 of these people came back to our special research clinics from time to time to be checked. We took blood samples and ran tests to see what was happening to their lipid levels. We also divided the patients into three more groups: 52 from each group either took choline or were checked for their progress without it for one year, 35 from each group stayed in the study for two years, and 28 from each group were on a three-year program.

The results were what research scientists call "promising," which means, "It looks like we're on the right track." At the end of the first year of the study, four of the fifty-two patients in the treated group had died—but ten of those in the control group had lost their lives.

That wouldn't have meant much if the trend had changed, but it didn't. In the two-year group, three of the thirty-five treated group patients had died, as compared to seven from the control group. And the three-year patients lost two from their treated group and three from their control group.

This pattern kept up during the second and third years, until the answer was too clear to be mistaken. After three years of keeping track, we found that 12 percent of the treated group had died, and 30 percent of the control group. Almost three times as many of the patients who had *not* received choline had died.

Of course, people can die for a lot of reasons, and no study can be called accurate unless all those possibilities are taken into account. We found that two patients in the treated group had died of causes that were not related to heart disease; this was true of four (twice as many) in the control group. But that still didn't change our results enough to make a significant difference. We were left with a 10-percent death rate in the treated group, compared to a 26-percent death rate in the control group.

A great deal of statistical analysis goes into a study like this, and Dr. Gonzalez and I spent a lot of time looking at our results from every possible angle, determined to be *sure* we had what we thought we had. We did. When we published the story of our work in the May, 1950, issue of the *American Heart Journal*, we wrote:

> The mortality rate [death rate] . . . appeared to be significantly reduced by the treatment with choline in this series of patients.
>
> These studies suggest that the lipotropic [lipid-lowering] agent choline is of value in the treatment of coronary arteriosclerosis and would appear to merit further trial and observation in this disease.

There's the phrase "further trial" again. In response to the need for further trials, a lot of other investigators did study choline, just as they had with lecithin.

Later the clues started coming in about choline's role as a neurotransmitter, and that created a tremendous amount of excitement in the scientific community—it was what we call a "major breakthrough." Some of this research resulted in a meeting in Belgium in 1976, in which an international group of doctors reported their findings about choline.

New Roles for Choline

What these doctors said at the international symposium filled an entire book, too technical to be understood by anyone other than their fellow scientists. But I can translate the essence of a couple of the chapters, just to make the point about how thoroughly choline has been tested and how good the results have been.

For example, V. Blaton, M.D., and his colleagues at the Simon Stevin Institute in Brussels, Belgium, gave ninety-two people injections of choline every day for two weeks. Examination of their blood showed that levels of LDL (the atherosclerosis-causing cholesterol) were lowered, and "25 percent of the lipoprotein patterns in Type II hyperlipidemia were normalized. . . . An average of 38 percent of the excess plasma cholesterol was eliminated."

Investigating another angle, J. Klemm, M.D., of Munich, Germany, gave 1,800 milligrams (almost 2 grams) of choline daily to twenty-six patients who suffered from poor blood circulation. After a month of this treatment, Dr. Klemm found that circulation was improved by 7 to 19 percent. He concluded that choline "causes a marked improvement of the blood-flow properties" in people with poor circulation. But he also noted that "in normal persons an increase in the blood flow was observed after the treatment."

One hindrance to normal circulation (and a contributor to atherosclerosis) is the tendency of platelets (blood cells) to clump together and form clots. Called "platelet aggregability," it is not the same thing as the tendency of platelets to stick to the walls of arteries—that's called "platelet stickiness." Choline helps to keep the platelets from clumping together. Their stickiness is affected by another ingredient of the Institute Formula, compounded plant extract (mucopolysaccharides). (More about that ingredient later.) The aggregability or clumping tendency was investigated by J. Schneider, M.D., G. Fuchs, M.D., and H. Kapronik, M.D., of Marburg, Germany, who gave 3 grams of choline daily to thirty-one patients who had Type II or Type IV hyperlipidemia.

"The total period of therapy was three and a half months," they wrote. "Already after eight weeks of treatment, a significant decrease of platelet aggregability was observed, whereas the number of platelets remained unchanged."

This illustrates the point that choline does not actually "thin" the blood. That is, it doesn't *remove* any of the platelets (which is good because they're necessary); it just helps to keep them from clumping together.

Memories Are Made of Choline

You could say that, at least in part, your memories are made of choline because without it you might not be able to recall them. That doesn't mean that a choline deficiency causes amnesia, or that administration of choline can cure it—there are many other factors involved. But, as science writer John Feltman reported in the April, 1979, issue of *Prevention*, "a study carried out by the National Institute of Mental Health indicates that a single dose of choline can significantly improve memory and recall, at least in normal, healthy individuals."

In this study, headed by N. Sitaram, M.D., people were able to memorize jumbled words more quickly after taking choline—and those who had the worst memories at the beginning of the study were the ones who improved the most. After this study was published in the scientific journal *Life Sciences* in 1978, Dr. Sitaram told Mr. Feltman, "Our studies show that choline has a weak to moderate memory-enhancement effect. It's not a robust effect, but it can be measured."

Scientists have not rushed to proclaim this effect of choline because it's still in the investigational stages. But in their own slow, careful way, investigators are trying to find out just *why* choline improves memory, how it works and how this knowledge can be used to help people. Most of the work so far has been done with experimental animals. A couple of preliminary reports were presented at the International Study Group on the Pharmacology of Memory Disorders Associated with Aging, held in Zurich, Switzerland, in April of 1981.

One of the speakers was Raymond T. Bartus, Ph.D., of Pearl River, New York, who said that his and other studies indicate that "under certain circumstances, choline can exert quite dramatic effects on memory performance." He had taken healthy young mice, given some of them diets that had been enriched with choline, and given others diets that were deficient in choline. After four and a half months, he subjected them to memory tests and compared their performances to those of (1) very young mice and (2) very old mice that had been fed regular diets.

He found that the choline-enriched mice performed as well as the very young ones, but the choline-deficient mice performed as poorly as the very old ones. "This study demonstrated," Dr. Bartus said, "that dietary manipulation of choline can significantly alter behavior in ways that are . . . similar to those occurring across the life span of the mouse. Thus, certain behavioral changes that occur with age might be modulated [lessened] through appropriate precursor control." By "precursor control" he meant control of substances in the body that serve as activators—in this case, choline.

In another study reported at the same meeting, Dr. Bartus told of elderly rats who had been fed a number of diet additives in an effort to improve their memories. Among these additives were choline alone and choline mixed with piracetam, a substance that helps the body to metabolize choline. The choline alone didn't fare very well in this test, but the choline mixed with piracetam produced "scores several times superior to those of rats given piracetam alone." This suggested, Dr. Bartus said, that "choline alone may not normally be sufficient to induce measurable behavorial improvement in aged subjects." But once the metabolism has been helped along by something such as piracetam, "this precursor [choline] may then exert reliable, positive effects."

One of Dr. Bartus's colleagues, Ronald F. Mervis, Ph.D., of Ohio State University, took Dr. Bartus's groups of mice and kept them on the choline-enriched or choline-deficient diets for six more months, then examined their brains. He found that the enriched mice had more connections between brain cells than either the deficient mice or ordinary mice. "This provides the first evidence of structural-behavioral alterations that can be directly attributed to dietary choline," he told the meeting in Zurich. As preliminary as these studies are, the implications are positive.

Does this mean that if you take choline you will not be forgetful in your old age? Not necessarily—but then again, maybe. The jury is still out. But so far choline has shown itself to be one of the most effective weapons we have against the deterioration that comes with old age. It is certainly good enough to have been included in the Institute Formula in a concentration of very high strength.

Ingredient Numbers 3 and 4: Phosphatidyl Inositol and Phosphatidyl Ethanolamine

I'm putting these two Institute Formula ingredients together because both of them are additional components of lecithin. They have been extracted and individually concentrated for the same reason choline was concentrated—to provide a much stronger extract than you could get in lecithin alone. Both are phospholipids, and both have the same characteristics and effects as lecithin. Although they have not been investigated much as individual substances, inositol is known as a vitamin of the B complex that is used in the growth of yeast; it also cures loss of hair in mice! (You learn the strangest things when you investigate human and animal chemistry; as far as I know, inositol will not cure baldness in people.)

But as a component of the Institute Formula it is just as valuable as any of the other ingredients in helping to lower lipid levels and forestall the degenerative changes that lead to arteriosclerosis, heart attack and stroke.

The Lecithin Controversy

Lecithin has gone through its shares of controversy since its introduction into medical practice in the 40s. While commercial preparation of it has become a major industry, and millions of people flock to health food stores to buy it and add it to their diets, there are some who think it's worthless, and still others who consider it harmful.

When something like that happens, you have to ask why? Probably the two biggest questions in research are Why? and Can you prove it? I've proved that lecithin can be helpful in lowering lipid levels, but other researchers believe they have proved that it won't. Why do we disagree? And why do some very intelligent, caring and highly educated scientists think lecithin is useless or harmful?

The answer is really very simple. It's that they are not aware that the results of lecithin tests depend upon the *type* of lecithin you use. To repeat myself for emphasis (and the point certainly is important enough to deserve repetition), choosing lecithin is like picking mushrooms in the woods—pick the right one and everything is fine; but pick the wrong one and you're in trouble.

The first error people make is selecting the wrong kind of lecithin in the wrong form. Manufacturers make a large variety of lecithin products through different processes of extraction, refinement and manufacture. This abundance of products hurts the public: When you can walk into a health food store and find a whole shelf full of bottles, jars and canisters simply labeled "lecithin," how do you know what you're getting? You don't—unless you make a point of looking for the word "soya" before "lecithin." If you see that, you know you're getting lecithin extracted from soybeans rather than egg yolks or any number of other saturated-fat sources. I also recommend that you use soya lecithin granules rather than tablets or capsules. Both the tablets and the capsules may include oil of unknown origin.

A second common mistake is the failure of many people—investigators and consumers alike—to realize that, whatever the extraction and manufacturing methods, there are some forms of lecithin that are downright dangerous to begin with because they are very high in saturated fat; the best example is the lecithin that occurs naturally in egg yolks. We know that fully or di-saturated fats readily attach themselves to the artery walls and contribute to the formation of the plaques and clots of atherosclerosis.

On the other hand, the lecithin extracted from soybeans is polyunsaturated, and is highest in choline, inositol and ethanolamine. This lecithin helps to carry cholesterol and related fats *out* of the arteries. Soya lecithin has been used by the Institute for Arteriosclerosis Research for more than thirty years in the prevention and treatment of atherosclerotic heart disease and premature aging.

There is a third, very important, and unfortunately very common oversight regarding lecithin: the amount you should take. The polyunsaturated fats in soya lecithin contain what we call "essential fatty acids" or "essential phospholipids" (EPL). These are exactly what their name implies: necessary for normal growth, nutrition and health. They contribute to the absorption of vitamins A and E. These essential phospholipids are supplied in the soya lecithin used at the Institute and included in the Institute Formula.

Be careful, though. Too much of a good thing is never a good idea, and scientists have learned that excessive use of polyunsaturated fats in the diet is unwise. The right amount is helpful; a lot is harmful—just as excessive use of any natural or normal components of foods may cause nutritional imbalance and metabolic harm.

These three factors, then, account for the controversy over lecithin's role in nutrition and preventive medicine. You have to use the right formulation, the right type and the right amount. In the Institute Formula, you get them all.

I have worked with a type of lecithin that contains at least 24 percent of the three ingredients just described: choline, inositol and ethanolamine. Continuous administration of this compound has resulted in a significant lowering of total blood cholesterol levels, triglyceride levels and VLDL levels, as well as the amounts of the greatest atherosclerosis producer of them all, the LDL cholesterol. What makes it even better is that the mixture also *raises* the amount of the protective cholesterol, HDL—the one that carries the harmful cholesterol out of the arterial cells and tissues. And to top it all off, it reduces the levels of blood fibrinogen, the substance that contributes to the clotting process. So this lecithin compound lowers the harmful cholesterol levels, elevates the protective cholesterol levels and lessens the tendency of the blood to create clots that can stick in narrowed arteries and slow or stop normal circulation.

Can I prove it? My colleagues and I have done so, again and again. As an example, let me tell you about five people who recently participated in a short-term clinical trial, taking a high potency soya lecithin that contained 34 percent choline, 20 percent inositol and 22 percent ethanolamine.

These five people took 30 grams of soya lecithin granules each day for twelve weeks. After six weeks, and again after the full twelve weeks, I tested their blood for cholesterol, triglycerides, HDL cholesterol, LDL and VLDL cholesterol and fibrinogen (the clotting factor). The averages of their results were:

- Total cholesterol levels fell from 290 to 208.
- Triglycerides fell from 138 to 103.
- HDL *rose* from 57 to 62.
- LDL fell from 150 to 121.
- VLDL fell from 96 to 28.
- Fibrinogen fell from 337 to 240.

These are excellent results! And this was only a short-term trial.

Only one of the five people had normal lipid levels at the beginning of the test. He was a 49-year-old male physician in very good health, and at the end of the test his lipid levels showed no significant change; that is, he started out normal and remained normal. This fact is very important because, as I've stated before, lower than normal lipid levels are dangerous. But if you're normal to begin with, soya lecithin will not significantly lower your lipid levels; it will help them to remain normal rather than rise above the normal range.

The other four subjects, all of whom had elevated lipid levels before the test, had been taking cholesterol-lowering drugs that had not produced good enough results. When they started taking the lecithin in this test, they stopped taking the other drugs, so there was no "enhancement" effect; the lecithin was acting alone in producing the good results we achieved.

All five subjects were following my low-fat, low-cholesterol diet before the test began. They continued to follow it during and after the test; none of them experienced any weight change, which was fine, since the diet they were using was a maintenance diet rather than one designed to either increase or reduce weight.

Let me tell you briefly what happened to the four people with elevated lipid levels in this test.

Louis, a 72-year-old man, was a chronic atherosclerotic, coronary-heart-disease patient with Type IV hyperlipidemia. He suffered from angina (chest pain), and from time to time his heart would flutter—that is, it would literally skip a beat (the medical name for this condition is "fibrillation"). He wasn't able to get around much because the slightest physical exertion would bring on the pain.

As you know, very advanced or terminal arteriosclerosis is irreversible. At Louis' age it was improbable that lecithin could completely clear the arteriosclerotic plaques in the arteries. In such a case, the objective of lecithin treatment was to halt the progress of the disease and to improve the individual's health and well-being.

The treatment worked. After the lecithin test Louis was able to tolerate exertion without pain; he could walk around and even perform light calisthenics. The quality of his life was definitely improved.

Then there was Angela, a 63-year-old woman who had the worst possible form of atherosclerosis in the arteries of her legs—atherosclerosis obliterans (meaning the arteries were obliterated by plaques) with claudication (pain and cramping when the patient tries to walk). Her condition was so serious that she had had bypass grafts in her left leg—surgery in which clear blood vessels are taken from another part of the body and sewn into the leg to create detours around the blocked arteries. Her right leg, unfortunately, was too far gone even for grafting, and had been amputated above the knee. She was barely able to move around, even with crutches, and she had anginal pain even at rest.

Twelve weeks of lecithin granules brought Angela a marked physical improvement. All her blood lipid levels were lowered significantly, and the pain at rest disappeared. She became able to walk around without pain, her energy increased, and her stamina (strength) and sense of well-being improved notably.

Caroline, aged 63, had arteriosclerosis in the arteries of her brain—extremely dangerous, since this condition leads to stroke. She had been declared "inoperable," the neurosurgeons stating they could not reach the obstructed arteries. On top of all that, she had high blood pressure and excessive levels of both total cholesterol and triglyceride. She suffered from "blackouts"—actual fainting spells—as well as terrible headaches and loss of some of her vision and hearing, all because of the blocked arteries in her brain. She had seriously thought of committing suicide.

Caroline represented what I would call our greatest success in this test; her response to the twelve weeks of lecithin was truly striking. Not only did her excessive lipid levels go down to normal, but her symptoms completely disappeared—and had not returned when she was examined again two years after the lecithin test. (If you're surprised that she was even alive two years later, you're in good company. Without the lecithin, she might not have been, or she might have been paralyzed by a stroke. Fortunately, we'll never know.) Caroline's sense of well-being was high (it had not existed at all before the test), and she said she felt she had been given "a new lease on life."

When you're working with people, every once in a while you're bound to run across somebody you just can't figure out—and our fifth patient, Marilyn, was one of those. All we really knew for sure about Marilyn was that she was 69 years old and had high blood pressure, excessive levels of cholesterol and triglyceride and coronary artery insufficiency. In addition to that she had a mixed bag of circulatory symptoms that were either vague or contradictory; it just wasn't possible to make a reliable clinical evaluation.

Nonetheless, we included her in the test group, which may have been a mistake. If her evaluation was unreliable, so was her compliance—we weren't at all sure that she was taking the daily dose of lecithin as instructed, and it seemed that she resented such a short-term trial period of treatment.

When we tried to evaluate the results of the test in her case, we did find that all three of her most important blood-clotting factors were significantly reduced. Yet her blood-lipid levels, measured at different times during the test, were sometimes reduced, sometimes unchanged, sometimes increased; we called them "mixed-up parameters." Unfortunately, such unpredictable and difficult to evaluate patients do come along every once in a while. However, when we knew that the patients were following the treatment schedule, the results of this test were consistently good.

Now a new form of lecithin/choline/inositol/ethanolamine has been incorporated into the Institute Formula, a compound that has not previously been available to the American public. It is more than double the potency and concentration of the strongest form of soya lecithin marketed up to now, and it has the added benefit of having been combined with the remaining six ingredients of the Formula.

Ingredient Number 5: Lethicon

This is a special form of lecithin, with a concentration of 55 to 95 percent choline, used as a stabilizer or regulator of lipids—especially in Europe, where it is known as "LipoStabil."

LipoStabil is not new. More than twenty years ago I was asked by its West German manufacturer to conduct a study of what they then called a "pure" form of choline—that is, 95 to 96 percent pure. The Institute scientists and I found that the pure choline, or LipoStabil, brought about a significant lowering of LDL and VLDL cholesterols (very desirable) and an increase in HDL cholesterol (very desirable, indeed). I kept the substance in mind as I went on to other studies.

At the 1976 meeting on choline in Belgium, A. M. Ehrly, M.D., and R. Blendin, M.D., of Frankfurt, Germany, reported that they had used LipoStabil in efforts to increase the efficient flow of blood. They found that injections of LipoStabil did, indeed, increase capillary flow rate, which is part of the microcirculation—the flow of particles too small to be seen with the naked eye. "Further studies" are again warranted, and are being carried out.

Meanwhile, LipoStabil or "lethicon," with all the benefits we have learned to expect from lecithin and choline, is an important part of the Institute Formula.

Ingredient Number 6: *Chondrus crispus* Extract

Several centuries ago, the people who lived on the rocky southern coast of Ireland discovered that the red seaweed growing along their shores was good for more than just its beauty. They mixed it with milk to make a rich pudding; no one knows who devised the recipe, but it was quite an innovation. I doubt that anyone then knew about the lipid-lowering abilities of the red seaweed, but they quickly discovered that it was a natural thickening agent—it could turn the thin liquid of milk into the creamy, rich substance of pudding.

Today we know that the same red seaweed grows along rocky coastlines in many other parts of the world as well—in Nova Scotia, Chile, Indonesia, Korea and, here in the United States, in Maine. It has several different names, which can be confusing if we don't sort them out right at the start.

The technical, biological name of the seaweed is *Chondrus crispus*. Some people call it Japanese seaweed because it was also discovered in Japan, others acknowledge the original discoverers by calling it Irish moss, and still others call it red seaweed because that's what it is. The Irish, speaking Gaelic in those days, called it *carraigeen*, and that has been modified to the modern-day name of carrageenan. If you're a label reader, you've probably seen "carrageenan" on a number of labels, since extracts of the seaweed are widely used as thickening agents and stabilizers in contemporary food processing.

It's very important to realize that there are an estimated 250 or more varieties of *Chondrus crispus*—and the possibilities for extraction are probably numberless. In the Institute Formula we use what we have found to be the most biologically potent extractions from all of them. To keep these straight I have named Ingredient Number 6 "*Chondrus crispus*" and Ingredient Number 7 "carrageenan extract." But they both come from the same general source, the red seaweed.

What's the difference between the two extracts? It's very complicated, based on their molecular structure, and would be baffling to anyone but a biochemist—and it wouldn't tell you what you need to know. I could, for example, break down and describe for you the molecular composition of a chair, but that wouldn't tell you how comfortable it is to sit in. Likewise, knowing that the difference between some red seaweed extracts depends on the amount of 3,6-anhydro-D-galactose each contains isn't going to tell you what the substance does for you. What's important is that the ingredients I call "*Chondrus crispus*" and "carrageenan extract" are both *beneficial* and *safe*.

Their safety, in fact, has been documented by the governmental watchdog agency, the Food and Drug Administration (FDA)—and if you've been watching the news lately you know how careful the FDA is about handing out its stamp of approval. These ingredients are listed in the FDA's book *Generally Regarded As Safe*, which scientists abbreviate GRAS. If a material is in GRAS, it's all right—and under "chondrus extract," the latest issue of GRAS says, "This substance is generally recognized as safe when used in accordance with good manufacturing practice."

For many years the harvesting of the red seaweed has been an annual event called "mossing"; in Canada it even has a regular season, regulated by the government, lasting from June to September. That makes it a natural occupation for students on summer vacation and lobster fishermen experiencing their slack season. Out they go in small boats, about two hours before low tide, scratching the seaweed off the rocks with long rakes that are specially built to capture only a certain amount, leaving behind the purple fronds that enable new moss to grow in the same spots. The Canadian government actually regulates the spacing of the teeth on the mossing rakes so that no one will take too much—mossing is an important industry in Canada.

The independent mossers sell their crop to processors who ship the raw product to drying and extracting plants. So important an industry is it that one processor, the Marine Colloids Corp., has distributed bumper stickers that are seen and believed in eastern Canada and Maine. They read: "Seaweed Power."

But, as is the case with so many natural resources, the demand for red seaweed has exceeded the supply. So what has the intrepid human mind done? Found a way to make more, of course. "What we've established is something very exciting and totally new," reported Louis Deveau, the former head of Marine Colloids Corp., in a descriptive booklet. On an "aquaculture research farm" in Nova Scotia, the firm has established "mechanically controlled pond cultures involving regulated seawater supply, the addition of nutrients, and stimulated water motion." Plans are underway for "a full commercial facility capable of producing a million pounds of Irish moss a year."

What does all this mean to you, the consumer interested in lowering his or her saturated-fat intake and preventing the degenerative diseases that lead to arteriosclerosis, heart attack and stroke? Simply that more red seaweed, *naturally grown*, will be available for extraction and inclusion in the Institute Formula at a reasonable cost. I emphasize "naturally grown" because I feel it important to stress that all the ingredients of the Institute Formula are completely natural plant products. Though some red seaweed is now cultivated on farms rather than growing spontaneously on rocks, no artificial additives or growth stimulants are used. Marine Colloids, for instance, has gone to a great deal of expense and carried out a great deal of research to make certain that the seaweed they produce is exactly the same as that harvested by vacationing students and lobster fishermen in Canada—but more of it is available, and not just between June and September.

Why are the seaweed extracts so important? Because they can *replace* cholesterol-rich substances in the thickening of foods, and they have lipid-lowering properties. In the special extractions formulated for the Institute Formula, red seaweed contributes to the reduction of dangerous fatty substances in your blood.

Ingredient Number 7: Carrageenan Extract

As mentioned earlier, "carrageenan" is another name for an extract of the *Chondrus crispus* seaweed. It's one that you may have seen on labels, since carrageenan has long been used in the food industry as a thickener and stabilizer. You're probably already eating a lot of carrageenan without even realizing it.

For example, have you ever wondered what holds your toothpaste together as it comes out of the tube? "Without minute amounts of carrageenan mixed in, the ingredients would be so runny they couldn't be squeezed out of the tube," the Marine Colloids booklet tells us. In chocolate milk, carrageenan keeps the milk and cocoa mixed so you don't have to stir constantly to keep the chocolate from settling to the bottom. In ice cream, carrageenan keeps the ingredients from separating as the delicious dessert melts. And in certain brands of "egg" custard, carrageenan is listed as a no-cholesterol replacement for eggs.

How does it work? Like a sponge, carrageenan soaks up water, forming a bulky but smooth gel in any liquid. It thickens, it stabilizes, it provides texture and body and it keeps ingredients from separating. Even your dog benefits from carrageenan—the moistness and freshness of canned dog food are maintained by this extract of red seaweed.

All this leads to an obvious question: "If I'm already getting carrageenan in so many of the foods I eat, why do I need more of it in the Institute Formula?" The answer is that carrageenan is used (as stated in the description of toothpaste) in "minute amounts" in everyday food processing. Its purpose in foods is to thicken and stabilize, not to nourish or lower lipids—in fact, I doubt that the people who originally discovered its thickening properties had any idea of the side benefits they were getting from carrageenan. But in the concentrated extracts used in the Institute Formula, you get the full benefit of the red seaweed substances: They stimulate repair and regeneration of cells, they provide sources of natural energy, they act as intestinal lubricants and (most important) they act as sponges—they pick up lipids, cholesterol and saturated fatty acids just as a sponge picks up water.

Also, about 10 percent of carrageenan is absorbed by the liver, where other agents are metabolized and fed into the bloodstream to act as protective and defensive agents against degenerative diseases.

Therefore, this beneficial product of seaweed, which you've been getting every time you eat ice cream or jelly or drink chocolate milk, is now provided in even greater (and certainly more healthful) concentrations in the Institute Formula.

Now you know how beneficial carrageenan is. But how safe is it? The following paragraph is quoted from a research paper published by Dimitri J. Stancioff, Ph.D., and Donald W. Renn, Ph.D., in the report of a symposium sponsored by the American Chemical Society in 1975:

> The safety of carrageenan as a food additive has been the target of many in-depth studies supported by government agencies here and abroad as well as by the various carrageenan producers. From the results of these studies, we can conclude that food-grade carrageenan— an isolated component of natural food products used extensively for over two centuries—has no adverse physiological effects, and that its safety in foods is assured.

Ingredient Number 8: Silicon

There's plenty of silicon already in your body—it is a trace mineral found in the connective tissues such as tendons, blood vessels and cartilage—but the older you grow, the less you have and the more you need.

In the Institute Formula, silicon performs much the same function that carrageenan carries out in chocolate milk: It binds the ingredients together so that they don't break into separate parts but stay together in a powder, capsule or tablet. However, we didn't put it in the Formula just to act as a powdered adhesive tape; silicon is part of the replacement-therapy function of the Formula.

Silicon is known to be an active component in the formation and maintenance of healthy connective tissues and bones—and also is known to slowly disappear as the body ages and the tissues and bones deteriorate. Investigators reporting in *Federal Proceedings* in 1974 stated that "the silicon content of the normal human aorta decreases considerably with age" and "the level of silicon in the arterial wall decreases with the development of atherosclerosis."

Logically, research efforts have been aimed at determining whether or not silicon added to the diet can replace the silicon lost during the aging process. So far, results indicate that it can.

One of the best known (and most controversial) of these studies was conducted by Klaus Schwarz, M.D., of the Department of Biological Chemistry at the UCLA School of Medicine in 1977. The conclusions of the study became known as the "hard-water theory," and a lot of skeptics thought it was nonsense to suggest that hard water contributed to health and was better for drinking than soft water. But Dr. Schwarz based his theory on the results of a heart-disease survey conducted in Finland between 1959 and 1974. It turned out that men in eastern Finland had twice as much heart disease (and related death) as did comparable men in the country's western end. The difference could not be explained by variations in controllable risk factors such as smoking and obesity.

Dr. Schwarz and his colleagues, testing the drinking water in both parts of the country, found that the level of silicon in the eastern (high-heart-disease) area was very low. But in the low-heart-disease western end, there was much more silicon in the hard water.

Pointing out that his was not the first study to indicate a strong protective quality in silicon-rich water, Dr. Schwarz stated: "The water factor, that is, the constituent of hard water that seems to exert an inhibitory effect on coronary heart disease, may be related to the amount of silicon supplied by water in different geological environments." In other words, the more silicon, the more protection against heart disease.

Dr. Schwarz also found a lot of silicon in foods that are high in dietary fiber—and fiber, as well as being highly desirable for digestive efficiency, is thought to lower blood cholesterol levels and therefore protect against heart disease.

But there are different kinds of fiber, and they occur in different foods. Some contain silicon, and some do not. Dr. Schwarz analyzed a number of different fiber foods for silicon content, and his results were reported in *Prevention* by Carl Sherman in 1978. "Sources of fiber with the demonstrated ability to lower cholesterol or prevent atherosclerosis—like alfalfa, rice hulls, pectin, and soybean meal—tested high in silicon," Mr. Sherman wrote. "Cellulose, which has no protective effect, tested low. And in wheat bran, where the results were uneven, Dr. Schwarz found uneven amounts of silicon."

Silicon, Dr. Schwarz and numerous other investigators concluded, is one very important reason why foods high in fiber are not only good but also essential for patients with heart disease. It stands to reason that they are just as important for *pre*-heart disease patients—that is, anyone who doesn't already have heart disease and doesn't want to get it.

So silicon exists in the Institute Formula for two purposes: as a binding and emulsifying agent, and as a replacement therapy for the silicon we lose naturally as we grow older.

Ingredient Number 9: Niacin

You've probably heard the word "niacin" often, since it is a member of the B-vitamin family and has been heavily publicized by advertisers promoting products in which it occurs. Multiple-vitamin compounds contain niacin in one form or another (you may have seen it as "niacinamide" or "nicotinic acid," and there are many other derivative forms). The U.S. Recommended Dietary Allowance (U.S. RDA) for niacin is 13 to 19 milligrams.

There has been a lot of argument among scientists about niacin, although it has been reported for decades as an effective agent for the reduction of LDL, VLDL, high cholesterol levels, total lipids and (to a lesser extent) triglycerides. It has been proposed and used as a treatment against coronary atherosclerosis, and it does have some significant effectiveness in that area. But its use has also resulted in some problems.

In 1974, the doctors' newspaper *Medical Tribune* reported on the work of Michael Rowe, M.D., and Michael Oliver, M.D., of the Royal Infirmary in Edinburgh, Scotland. In an effort to lower free fatty acid levels, the doctors had given a derivative of nicotinic acid to forty patients immediately after they had suffered myocardial infarction (heart attack). They found that treated patients had significantly fewer arrhythmias (heart flut-terings) in the first few hours after their heart attacks than did patients who didn't receive nicotinic acid. This, they reasoned, was due to the fact that free fatty acid levels shoot up right after a heart attack, a sudden increase that has been connected to potentially fatal complications. Drs. Rowe and Oliver based their experiment on the long-standing belief that nicotinic acid has a definite lipid-lowering effect. But they ran into problems with other effects for which it's also famous: In large doses, niacin is known to create some very unpleasant side effects, including nausea, vomiting, flushing and itching. Yet, if a med-icine can save your life when you've just had a heart attack, the uncomfortable side effects do not seem important.

On the basis of this study, "It is planned to add the new treatment to the equipment of the city's [Edinburgh] mobile coronary care units," Dr. Rowe was quoted as saying. "We are going to try to get to patients much sooner, so that we can begin lowering their free fatty acid levels before they leave their homes."

The use of niacin may be very good for people who have had heart attacks within the last hour, but what does it have to do with you? I use the example simply to point out that the lipid-lowering ability of niacin is so well established that it can be used in emergency situations as well as in long-term treat-ment and in prevention. You have to give a great deal of it to someone who's just had a heart attack, and you have to do it fast. However, in smaller amounts, over long periods of time, niacin still lowers lipid levels.

As I mention again and again (with good reason), the *amount* of a substance can make all the difference as to how well it does the job you want it to do, and whether or not it does other things (that you don't want it to do) at the same time. The effectiveness of niacin has been proven in studies such as the one carried out in 1975 by Ralph Brattsand, M.D., of Sweden, that showed a 20 percent reduction in plasma cho-lesterol in rabbits fed niceritrol (a niacin derivative).

In people, "Niacin is an effective hypolipidemic agent when administered in doses exceeding its daily requirement as a vitamin," wrote Robert I. Levy, M.D., of the National Heart, Lung and Blood Institute in the *Journal of the American Medical Association* in 1976. "Within four to six hours it depresses plasma triglyceride concentrations by reducing VLDL synthesis. The drug also has an indirect lowering effect on IDL [intermediate-low-density lipoprotein] and LDL levels, which occurs only after several days."

But Dr. Levy devoted several paragraphs of his article to descriptions of unpleasant side effects, including flushing of the skin, itching, nausea and problems with liver function and blood-sugar levels. He warned his physician readers, "Great caution is therefore advised in considering use of the drug in patients with liver disease, diabetes, or gout."

Remember, however, that he said, "doses exceeding its daily requirement as a vitamin." As I've already mentioned, the U.S. RDA for niacin is 13 to 19 milligrams. In his article, Dr. Levy explained that he was referring to doses of 100 milligrams a day, which "can be increased 300 milligrams per day every four to seven days for a maintenance dose of 3 to 9 grams per day. The usual adult dose is 1 gram three times a day." Since 1,000 milligrams equals 1 gram, that means 3,000 milligrams per day—or over 150 times the RDA!

Does that mean that you can't get a lipid-lowering effect from niacin unless you take enough to make you sick? Not necessarily. In the amount we use in the Institute Formula (50 milligrams, or 1½ times the U.S. RDA), niacin acts mainly as a catalyst—that is, an activator or booster—to the other nine ingredients. The amount is small enough to give you the benefit without the side effects, and the vitamin is well diluted since it is acting in concert with the other nine ingredients. I don't suggest that you take large doses of niacin by itself; in the Formula you get a safe amount that helps the total mixture to strengthen your fight against degenerative diseases leading to arteriosclerosis, heart attack and stroke.

Chapter 5

THE INSTITUTE FORMULA: INGREDIENT NUMBER 10—MPS

Scientific research is a lot like a treasure hunt or a good detective story, except that it takes a great deal longer. There are clues to follow—false clues that lead to disappointment and frustration as well as good clues that raise your spirits and keep you going—periodic encouragements and blind alleys. Every once in a while there's the thrill of finding something that tells you, yes, all the hard work was worth it and you've been on the right track all along. That is what we mean when we use a word that has become overworked lately but still carries its special, uplifting meaning: breakthrough.

The discovery of the components of Ingredient Number 10 and how they work was definitely a breakthrough. It made sense. It was based on sound, proven medical history and cautious, logical theory. It was just too logical to be ignored. And it happened a long time ago.

Nature is certainly the world's greatest balancing act, which is why life as we know it has managed to survive. If everything in nature were positive—if we had no weaknesses or illnesses and death were unknown—this planet would have crowded itself out of existence millions of years ago. On the other hand, if only negative forces existed, or if they were allowed to prevail, plant and animal life would never have survived the Stone Age. But strengths balance weaknesses, births balance deaths, and even though individuals come and go, life (so far) wins out in the long run. That may read like a bit of heady philosophy, but it's actually just an interpretation of what science knows to be one of nature's extraordinary phenomena: To all natural biologic properties there are counterbalancing properties with opposing biologic actions.

Does that mean that for every bad biologic action there is a good biologic action of equal strength? Not exactly—if nature were that mathematically precise, someone probably would have figured it all out centuries ago. But it does mean that, in living tissues, human tissues in particular, where there are destructive, degenerative forces, there are also *re*generative, reparative forces opposing them.

What it boils down to is that we have natural weapons against degenerative disease, and they have been provided for us by nature. The treasure hunt begins when we realize that they exist and set out to find them—and to use them for our benefit.

We know, for example, that the heart, blood vessels and other vital organs are made up of connective tissues that maintain their structure and function. These are the good forces. They are opposed by the bad forces: enzymes, hormones and hormonelike signalling agents that permit degeneration and disease. They are also opposed by outside agents—in the case of arteriosclerosis and heart disease, these consist of saturated fats and lipids. The good forces have to be very strong, indeed, to survive against both internal and external opponents.

For a long time, the only good forces we had were the internal ones that nature gave us. Then, as scientists learned more about the structure and function of the body, we began to provide ourselves with some external weapons as well. Among the most important of these was *knowledge*—the knowledge that we could cut down the power of the external bad forces simply by controlling what we eat and the amount of exercise we get. We also devised medicines to help us when the bad forces got the upper hand. But still we were faced with a very powerful opponent that struck at many of us through heredity: deficiencies.

A deficiency is an uncontrollable risk factor in heart disease. As I have pointed out in earlier chapters, some people are born with a tendency to hyperlipidemia or with an inability to handle the fatty content of food. And even normal persons can be overwhelmed by excessive amounts of saturated fats in the diets popular in Western countries. Lecithin, choline, niacin, all the ingredients in the Institute Formula, are powerful weapons against deficiencies and heavy attacks by external lipids. But the real strength of the Formula lies in an ingredient that has been around for a long time but only recently has received recognition as the tremendous regenerative weapon it is. Meet Ingredient Number 10: a category of connective-tissue components known as mucopolysaccharides or glycosaminoglycans.

Both these words are the tongue-twisters you can expect from scientific terminology. Why the scientific community, already overburdened with mile-long words, invented two such unpronounceable terms for the same thing is one of those mysteries I don't bother trying to solve. It's much easier just to use the accepted abbreviation for mucopolysaccharides: MPS.

What are MPS, and how can they help you to prevent the degenerative diseases that lead to arteriosclerosis, heart attack and stroke?

They are primarily carbohydrates linked to protein. I say "primarily" because there are many MPS from many sources, and they have many variations in structure. But for this study it is most important to know that the MPS are naturally occurring components of connective tissue that exist in both animals and plants. The MPS that you get in Ingredient Number 10 of the Institute Formula—compounded plant extract—are derived, as the name suggests, from plants.

This ingredient is a grab-bag of good biologic elements from the same types of seaweed that give us the *Chondrus crispus* and carrageenan extracts. In fact, one of the biggest problems I had with this ingredient was figuring out what to call it. It's a mixture, actually a very complicated mixture, of MPS substances with convoluted technical names only a graduate biochemist could love. Since the final ingredient is a compound of extracts from plants, I called it compounded plant extract, or CPE.

Remember that there are more than 250 varieties of red seaweed. CPE is a mixture drawn from the best of the naturally occurring anti-degenerative, anti-aging components of carefully selected varieties of seaweed. It has the sponging effect of *Chondrus crispus*, a binding effect and an anti-atherogenic and anti-coagulant effect. Best of all, it is a natural replacement therapy—it replaces missing MPS for people who do not have enough, and strengthens natural MPS for people who do have sufficient amounts.

The MPS in Nature

Just what are the MPS, and what do they do? These questions were answered by Orville Miller, Ph.D., of the School of Pharmacy, University of Southern California, in 1973. Writing in the book *Applied Nutrition in Clinical Practice,* Miller quoted the definition of "mucopolysaccharide" he had found in a medical dictionary: "Thick gelatinous material found in many places in the body. It glues cells together, lubricates joints, and is found in blood-group substances."

Explaining what the MPS do, Dr. Miller wrote:

> *Mucopolysaccharides play a major role in the structural integrity of all body tissues and are largely responsible for the form and organization of the human system as components of connective tissue. They have aptly been described as the "glue of life." They are involved in transfer of electrolytes and nutrients through cell walls. Mucopolysaccharides occur in the organic matrix of bone and teeth and function in both a structural and nutritional capacity. They are also largely responsible for the elasticity of skin and of blood vessels.*

The key words are "elasticity of blood vessels." The role of MPS in maintaining that elasticity is the reason for the work I've done with MPS and the reason they are so important to the Institute Formula.

The arteries are the biggest of the blood vessels. When their walls become clogged with atherosclerotic plaques, the arteries *lose* their elasticity and become hard—which is why we call arteriosclerosis "hardening of the arteries." Because MPS contribute to the elasticity of the blood vessels, the introduction of supplementary MPS in the form of the Institute Formula helps to maintain their natural, healthy flexibility.

On the subject of deficiency diseases, Dr. Miller pointed out that "many diseases are associated with changes in the mucopolysaccharide content of the tissues involved," listing atherosclerosis along with rheumatoid arthritis, asthma, emphysema and others. "Aging," he said, "if it can be considered a disease, is accompanied by changes in mucopolysaccharide content of many tissues, both in kind and quantity." Of course, aging itself is not technically a disease since it is a natural event that no one can escape, but we now know that we can prevent or lessen the degenerative changes that afflict so many people with the passing of the years. Replacing some of the lost MPS is one of the ways to do that.

Later in his writing, Dr. Miller arrived at the point (in 1973) that had been the basis of this particular breakthrough, and had been my theory as far back as 1942. "If a lack of appropriate mucopolysaccharide can cause disease," he suggested, "it should be possible to treat disease by administration of mucopolysaccharide or precursors needed for biosynthesis. A review of the literature reveals that this is indeed possible and may well represent the next major advance in medical science."

Dr. Miller's statement was right on target. Among the literature that he cited was a paper I had published in 1965—a paper that represented scientific studies dating back to 1942.

The Early Studies

Back then, I had begun my work on MPS with a special form taken from the aortas of calves. As you have seen, early in my career I adhered to the belief that replacement of deficient substances was a valid and effective form of therapy. I knew that this form of MPS (which had been described originally in 1861 but not really investigated until the late 30s) was either deficient or abnormal in arteriosclerotic arteries studied by other investigators. Therefore, it was my theory that replacing the missing MPS should help restore those arteries to normal.

The theory was based on logic and the results of earlier studies using replacement therapy (notably the liver juices I've already described), but I still had to prove it. As usual, that took a very long time.

Between 1942 and 1955, I treated a total of 134 arteriosclerosis patients with this form of MPS, giving the extracts to some by mouth and to others through injections. Ninety-nine of these people had coronary arteriosclerotic heart disease (group 1), 29 had arteriosclerosis of the cerebral (brain) arteries (group 2), and 6 had hardening of the arteries of the legs (group 3). Fifty-six of the patients in group 1 took the special MPS extract for three years; the other 43 in group 1 and most of those in group 2 took it for three months; and the 6 patients in group 3 took it for six months.

The results were more than good, they were marvelous, and spurred me on to much more extensive work with MPS. In group 1, 74 percent of the patients improved on MPS; in group 2 the improved rate was 77 percent; and in group 3 it was best of all, an 80 percent improvement!

After that early success I went on to much more thorough research into the benefits of MPS, doing a great deal of work with animals as well as human patients. In 1963, my coinvestigators and I published the results of a study done with cells in the laboratory, a type of study which is like taking a clock apart and examining each of the pieces individually to find out exactly *why* your repair method works as well as it does.

The lab work was done with cells taken from the inside walls of the aortas of chicks. After loading these cells with a "diet" of cholesterol, we then fed them the test mucopolysaccharide medium, and found that significant decreases in lipid content resulted. This, I wrote with great satisfaction, "confirms studies indicating that total lipids and cholesterol are significantly reduced per unit volume of cells when very small amounts of mucopolysaccharide, in the form of calf aorta extracts, are added to the cultures." And that wasn't all: Two years later my colleagues and I were able to report that "under specific conditions, MPS will act as a growth-stimulating agent," and "it may be a metabolic agent in the regulation of cell processes."

Meanwhile, other scientists had also been working with MPS, especially in Japan. In 1959, S. Ohdoi, M.D., of Tokyo reported that MPS derived from shark cartilage appeared to reduce the rate at which atheromatous lesions formed in the aortas of cockerels. And Katsumi Murata, M.D., Ph.D., who has done a lot of work with me at the Institute for Arteriosclerosis Research, published in 1962 a report of his work with rabbits.

Dr. Murata injected highly sulfated MPS into the rabbits' veins, and found that it reduced concentrations of total lipids and cholesterol; therefore, it lessened the severity of arteriosclerosis. After his work on rabbits, he teamed up with Dr. Y. Oshima to test whether MPS would benefit people.

Drs. Murata and Oshima gave 1.5 grams of MPS powder (from shark cartilage) by mouth to people who had excessively high cholesterol levels, as well as to some whose cholesterol levels were normal. In the normal subjects, nothing happened—cholesterol levels remained normal. But in the hypercholesterolemic people, two to four weeks of taking powdered MPS brought about an average 18 percent reduction in total serum cholesterol.

That was just the beginning. Knowing that squirrel monkeys get and suffer from arteriosclerosis in very much the same way humans do, we fed a cholesterol-and-butter diet to sixty-five of these animals for nine months. I also gave MPS to selected groups of them. "Monkeys treated with MPS and fed the cholesterol-butter diet showed statistically significant reductions of serum total lipid levels and aorta lipid levels when compared to control groups on the cholesterol-butter diets," I reported. "The acid mucopolysaccharides may be an effective preventive agent in the treatment of experimentally induced atherosclerosis."

When I reported on this study at the 1965 meeting of the American Heart Association's Council on Arteriosclerosis, the *New York Times* ran an article on it very cautiously suggesting that my co-workers and I might have something important. The article that appeared in the *Times* said:

> *The work that produced MPS was based initially, Dr. Morrison explained in an interview, on the concept that normal tissues contain various regulatory substances that help keep them normal.*
>
> *Thus, blood vessels might contain a substance that regulates fat metabolism, thereby inhibiting the development of fatty atherosclerotic deposits in the walls of those structures, which block them and lead to cardiovascular trouble.*
>
> *If such a substance could be found, administration of it to persons susceptible to the development of atherosclerosis might prevent the disease.*

Such a substance *had* been found, but the public as well as the scientific community was characteristically slow to recognize it and reluctant to accept it. Three more years passed before the *Journal of the American Geriatrics Society* published my report of a second study, on human subjects.

Over a period of one to two years, I had given MPS in powder or tablet form to 60 patients who had proven coronary arteriosclerotic heart disease, and had compared them to another 60 patients who did not get MPS, a total study population of 120. Among the 60 untreated patients, thirteen coronary incidents occurred, and two of these resulted in the patients' deaths. But in the treated group, only one coronary incident (a fatal heart attack) occurred.

In 1969 I published a follow-up report in the *Journal of the American Geriatrics Society* stating that by then a total of twenty-one coronary incidents had occurred in the control (untreated) group (four of these patients died), but only three of the sixty treated patients had suffered similar attacks. "The ratio of 21:3 for coronary episodes in the MPS group versus the non-

MPS group warrants further studies with acid mucopolysaccharides," I concluded. (There's that phrase "warrants further studies" again.) But this time I went further and explained something I had learned from motion picture films and microscopic photographs of animal arteries: It appeared that an important reason for the action of this particular mucopolysaccharide lay in electrically charged forces. "The electro-negative charges on blood platelets and cells prevent aggregation, adhesion, or 'stickiness,' thereby preventing or delaying thrombus [clot] formation," I wrote. "At the same time, electro-negative repellent charges are exerted upon the vascular endothelium lining the artery wall."

What does that mean? The phenomenon is like magnetism. If you hold opposite poles of a magnet together, they stick. But if you hold two poles of the same charge together, they not only don't stick, they push away, or repel each other. Something in MPS, it seemed, helped the blood platelets and cells to develop the same "anti-magnetic" force against the walls of the arteries—which meant the blood kept on circulating instead of sticking to the arteries or clotting. When we gave oral MPS to patients who had angina pectoris (chest pain caused by narrowed arteries), it took longer for their blood to clot than it had before the treatment.

First Line of Defense

In my 1969 article I described MPS as the arterial wall's first line of defense against the invasion of foreign or noxious substances. "The primary action of certain acid mucopolysaccharides involves repair, regeneration, and growth of normal new tissues," I wrote, and I had the statistics to prove it.

Many of these statistics—and conclusions—about MPS had come from experimental studies done on animals. In 1966, for example, I published the results of a research project in which rats had been fed diets heavy in cholesterol and had also been subjected to very high doses of X rays. A few years earlier, other investigators had proved that extreme exposure to X rays would increase both the incidence and the severity of atherosclerotic lesions in these animals. That gave us a way of creating test subjects much more quickly.

Once we had a good supply of atherosclerotic rats, we gave some of them MPS by injection, while others got it by mouth. Still others were injected with a plain saline solution.

We found that taking MPS by mouth produced positive results. The rats who got it by injection remained seriously affected by lipid deposits in their arteries, and the same was true of those who got the saline solution. But the rats who received MPS by mouth "exhibited a striking reduction in both the incidence and extent of lipid deposition in the coronary arteries."

When we examined the hearts of these rats, we found lipid deposition in fewer than 10 percent of them, and what we did find was considered "minimal." The amount found in the hearts of the other rats, however, was enough to be called "marked."

Later we tried oral MPS on rats that had been rendered atherosclerotic by diets that contained high levels of cholesterol plus extreme overdoses of vitamin D_2. Of the thirty-four rats on this diet, thirty-three had severe lesions of the coronary arteries within six weeks.

We gave the same diet *plus MPS* to thirty-six other rats. Lesions of the aorta developed in only five of these rats, and only six had lipid-containing coronary lesions.

A New Partner

From 1962 to 1968, Dr. Katsumi Murata took a leave of absence from the University of Tokyo and came to California to work with us at the Institute for Arteriosclerosis Research. He helped us with our work on squirrel monkeys, rats and rabbits, and we found that the way MPS was given produced different results in different species of animals. Whereas injection did nothing for the rats, it worked on the monkeys, giving us "clear evidence of prevention of aortic atherosclerosis."

We reported these findings in a journal called *Experimental Medicine and Surgery* in 1967, explaining that "we have considered the possibility that MPS may act therapeutically upon the connective tissue of the artery wall to account for its antiatherogenic properties in experimental atherosclerosis." We also suggested that "certain mucopolysaccharides may have value in the treatment and/or prevention of atherosclerosis in man."

At that time I was also working with B. H. Ershoff, Ph.D., and P. R. Rucker, M.S., on determining what effect MPS would have on the formation of blood clots. This study was done with rabbits.

We compared MPS with heparin, a drug that has a long and respectable reputation in preventing blood clots. It is often given to people who have had heart attacks to prevent a second attack.

Our study with rabbits showed that MPS did the job just as well as heparin, but that the good effect lasted longer—five *days* as compared to five hours with heparin. We measured the effectiveness of these agents by determining how long it took for a thrombus (clot) to form in the blood—the longer the better, up to a point.

One problem with heparin is that its effect doesn't last very long. About five hours or more after a patient receives a safe and effective dose, he needs another one to maintain the anti-clotting quality of his blood. So doctors have to give heart patients a lot of heparin and do it often, which leads to another problem with the drug—after a while it can build up, make the blood too thin, and cause a hemorrhage. Obviously, people who take heparin have to be watched very carefully, and that means a lot of time spent in the doctor's office.

We found that MPS acts much more slowly. Twelve hours after the first dose, when the heparin-treated rabbits needed another injection, the MPS-treated rabbits still had clotting times four times longer than those before treatment. Even forty-eight hours—two full days—after the first dosage, their clotting times were still three times longer than at the beginning. MPS was obviously a much-longer-acting clot preventer.

We suggested, as usual, that more tests should be done to see how well this principle works in humans. Then we went ahead and did more advanced work of our own with dogs (it's not easy to get permission to try new drugs on people). The dog study, published in 1970, produced the same results: MPS lasted much longer than did heparin.

Therapeutic Applications

By 1977, enough experiments had been done to convince me (and a lot of other investigators) that MPS had an important role to play in combating heart disease. But we had to convince many other people of the value of MPS. Doubts were raised by the fact that other investigators had tried it and found either no results or serious side effects. Naturally, they weren't about to endorse it.

However, there was a very good reason why our MPS worked, and theirs didn't. In 1977, in *Folia Angiologica*, an international medical journal, I pointed out:

> *The properties of MPS hinge upon a highly critical factor. This is the process of MPS manufacture, which can or cannot preserve the high biologic potency re-*

*sulting from gentle extraction of the acid mucopolysac-
charide, instead of the harsh chemical processes often
used commercially to produce a faster, less expensive
and thus monetarily salable product.*

That's an old story, brought home by the proverb, Haste
makes waste. Cheap, fast methods of production produce a
cheap, chemically contaminated MPS of poor quality. The same
is true of so many products today. If you interfere too much
with nature and come up with a cheap, artificial version of
anything, you're going to have a very inferior product. When
the product is something that affects health, the result can even
be dangerous.

At the Institute we take great pains to use the resources
nature has given us, staying away from the chemicals and additives that our bodies were never intended to consume. Other
laboratories were working with MPS that had lost its anti-clotting ability through chemical processing. Some of the mucopolysaccharides actually *caused* clotting, and as a result got a
very bad press.

Klaus Schwarz, M.D., who has written much on the need
for adequate silicon in the prevention of heart disease, found
that MPS from the Institute was high in silicon. But harsh chemical processing may remove much of the silicon from the MPS
used by other scientists.

All these factors contribute to conflicting results and make
it difficult, if not impossible, to convince the authorities that
properly produced MPS is a truly valuable weapon in the fight
against heart disease.

But the MPS contained in the Institute Formula under
the collective name compounded plant extract (CPE) have proven
themselves time and again to be effective in preventing the
degenerative changes that lead to arteriosclerosis, heart attack
and stroke. Their anti-lipidemic effect is well known, and they
have been extracted and compounded into a concentration that
provides the very best the plant world can currently offer us
in our fight to counteract the debilitating effects of aging. As
Dr. Miller wrote in his article on mucopolysaccharides:

*Use of these materials in their crude, natural state re-
quires a substantial dosage. Fractionation of several of
these items has produced useful clinical products of moderate dosage. Eventual isolation and production of the*

essential components should finally introduce the era of curative medicine.

In the Institute Formula, I believe this goal has been reached.

Ingredient Numbers 1 through 10: New Hope

There you have it: the Institute Formula. It is the result of years of work with each of the ingredients alone, with various combinations, and with the final "recipe" of the ten ingredients I have just described. For the first time, to my knowledge, we have a synergistic mixture of ten natural substances, each of which has been scientifically proven, over and over again, to be effective against the production and occurrence of degenerative diseases leading to arteriosclerosis, heart attack and stroke. It is an innovation and, yes, a breakthrough.

After the extensive testing I've described, you may wonder whether the final formula, with all ten ingredients together, has also been tested. The answer is yes, of course it has. But in this case I don't have a number of published reports to quote because the work has been done privately at the Institute for Arteriosclerosis Research in California, and this book is the first publication of the results. You have in your hands the first release of what has truly been a Secret Formula.

Why secret? Because I didn't want it to be known until I was positive, beyond any doubt, that it was as good as I expected it would be, that it was the best it could be, and that no harmful side effects could occur. Also, I did not want a lot of inferior imitations to appear throughout the world as was the case with various of the Institute's other discoveries.

As I have explained, the extraction processes we use must be extremely precise in order to produce ingredients that will give the desired results without causing any bad side effects. Also—especially in the case of niacin—the amounts must be precise. It's unfortunate but true that there are many people who will jump on any bandwagon that sounds profitable and create imitations of a good thing. Some of these imitations might be worthless, while others could conceivably be harmful. So I have kept the Institute Formula to myself until I had it perfected—and now I am gratified to be able to present it to the world in the natural, pure form in which it can do the most good.

It was about fifteen years ago that I realized how logical it was, in view of the demonstrated success of each of these ingredients against degenerative diseases, to combine them into a single entity. Each of these substances had been proven effective by numerous investigators and research scientists, then investigated and reinvestigated. Now the time had come to bring about a merger—to use them all together at their highest level of effectiveness. In the Institute Formula they are used at their highest biologic potency, in the most natural way and the safest way.

Of course you may wonder how I determined how much of each ingredient to put into the final formula. The answer is: by trial and error, by clinical observation, by studying the evidence gained from innumerable tests. I was like a chef creating a vital recipe—a recipe for life. Although I certainly did not work alone, this is one case in which too many cooks did not spoil the broth. All the scientists who worked at and with the Institute for Arteriosclerosis Research made invaluable contributions, and we received a lot of indirect help from the work of other investigators whose reports we read in the medical and scientific journals. The full roster of the Institute Formula Team appears in the front of this book.

We first began to use the combination of ingredients— the recipe called the Institute Formula—clinically in 1966, but the most intensively measured and studied tests began in 1975. Although the results were conclusive and tremendously exciting, I was warned not to publish the results of these studies then because the final formula would be stolen, imitated and exploited. So the results, as well as the details of the studies themselves, were kept confidential until now.

The primary study of the final formula was done at the Institute for Arteriosclerosis Research in California with sixty-five patients, all of whom had advanced coronary heart disease. At the same time, my colleague in London, Carl H. Goldman, M.D., was conducting a similar study with fifty-three patients from his private practice. After three years, Dr. Goldman and I got together to compare our results, and it was a triumphant day, indeed. Not only were the results of the two studies almost exactly the same, they proved beyond any doubt that we had something truly effective on our hands.

My group of sixty-five patients received the formula in tablet, capsule or powdered form, with an average dosage of 8 grams a day, given in two 4-gram dosages. The powder was given as an additive to food or drink—most of the patients like to sprinkle it over cereal or mix it up in a blender with a favorite drink. Although different people took the formula for different periods of time, the average duration of treatment was 7½ months.

Unfortunately, one of the sixty-five patients had to drop out of the study because of nausea and vomiting after ingesting the formula. This is the same type of food sensitivity that some people have to the ingredients of the formula—vitamins, minerals and seaweed derivatives. On the plus side, however, the percentage of people in the general population who have this sort of sensitivity is very low; in my series, one out of sixty-five constitutes 1.5 percent.

I lost another four patients because of travel problems— they lived too far away to continue the program after they had been discharged from the hospital. So after starting out with sixty-five, I had sixty left on whom to judge the results of the new formula.

Out of sixty patients, forty-five, or 75 percent, improved on this treatment. Another fifteen (25 percent) remained the same. Not one experienced a worsening of symptoms.

What symptoms are we talking about? The patients reported lessened angina (chest pain), lessened incidence of dizziness, lessened pain in the legs (caused by poor circulation in clogged arteries) and increased tolerance to exercise. Medical examinations showed improvement in the abnormalities seen on their electrocardiograms and improvements in their heart rates and rhythms. This is particularly significant when you consider the fact that all of these patients had severe, advanced, proven coronary heart disease that had not responded to conventional therapy.

Meanwhile, in England, Dr. Goldman was having similar good results with his fifty-three patients. At the end of the study period he reported that forty-three (81 percent) had shown marked, moderate or mild improvement, and nine (17 percent) had stayed the same. One patient (2 percent), an 81-year-old man, had died while attempting to perform vigorous physical exercise.

When you add Dr. Goldman's statistics and mine together, you get 113 patients (after subtracting the 5 who dropped out of my group and were not counted in the totals). Of these, 88 (78 percent) improved after taking the Institute Formula, 24 (21 percent) stayed the same and 1 (nine-tenths of 1 percent) died. These remarkable results are even more impressive when you compare them to statistics published in the medical literature about patients with the same type and degree of coronary heart disease.

For example, Dr. Goldman and I cited a study of 2,020 patients in Utah who had suffered myocardial infarctions (heart attacks) and been treated in hospitals. Of the 2,020, 379 (19 percent) died in the hospital under conventional treatment. Of the 1,641 who survived long enough to leave the hospital, 22 percent died within the next three months, also on conventional treatment. After that, the death rate was 5 percent yearly for the next five years.

Of course, all is not perfect, in nature or in man's activities. In my group of sixty-five patients, with its zero death rate (the death rate is considered to be the best measurement of a formula's effectiveness, in my view and also in that of the scientific community), there were two patients who suffered nonfatal myocardial infarctions. One of these people was the victim of one of the most severe cases of heart disease and heart failure I have ever seen; the other was a man who went without the formula for three months, at which time his infarction occurred. These two cases had to be included in the study in order to make it absolutely complete, with the negative as well as the positive results. So the negative result in my study of sixty patients was two heart attacks, or 3 percent.

In spite of these two cases, the results were so overwhelmingly positive that I considered the time right to bring the formula to the public. In the report of our combined study (as yet unpublished in the medical literature), Dr. Goldman and I wrote:

> *All these natural substances, when combined in a single synergistic blend, are illustrative of the euclidean theorem that the whole is greater than the sum of its parts. In the same way, the entire Institute Formula had demonstrated itself to be more highly effective in this total formulation than has been found and described by scientific publications in previous years.*

You can see, then, why I suggest you take the Institute Formula as a whole rather than simply using food supplements such as lecithin, choline, niacin and silicon. Of course, you could derive health benefits if you did just that. But, as you know from reading this book, the ingredients in the Institute Formula act together, and many of them are special, high-potency forms of lecithin, choline and MPS—forms that no one can duplicate without a laboratory and tremendous expertise. So, to ensure that you can get it in its purest, safest—and most potent and effective—form, the Institute continually tests the supplies used in the Formula. Also, I have personally licensed several commercial organizations to prepare and distribute the Institute Formula to the general public.* I want you to know, too, that I derive no financial benefit whatsoever from this product. All proceeds that I receive from the Institute Formula—and from this book—go directly to the Institute for Arteriosclerosis Research (from which I do not receive a salary or any type of remuneration) to further its ongoing research into the causes, prevention and potential successful treatments of circulatory disease.

Individual Differences

Of course, the results from taking the Institute Formula will not be the same for everyone. I have already pointed out that advanced arteriosclerosis cannot be reversed, although its progress can be slowed or stopped, and the person who already has this disease can feel better and live longer even though damage has already been done. But the younger and healthier a person is when he begins to supplement his diet with the Institute Formula, the more it will be able to help him—and the longer he will be able to enjoy a rich and healthy life without the handicaps of degenerative diseases.

You know, of course, that you can never expect a miraculous response to any medication, substance, preventive or therapeutic agent just by popping a pill into your mouth every once in a while. In a preventive program in particular, results may not be obvious—the result, after all, is what *doesn't* happen rather than what does. It is imperative that where obvious need exists for such a substance (and the tragic rate of heart disease in this country is "obvious need" enough for me), large, adequate amounts of the compound must be taken over long periods of time. And "adequate amounts" will not be the same for everyone. One must cut the cloth according to the pattern, or "tailor" the amounts given according to the individual's needs.

Just as there are no two fingerprints exactly alike, so there are differences in the needs and responses of individuals to anything, including a food or a medicine. The amounts used fall into a spread or range of response of which a mean or average is employed to determine the proper dosage for the majority of people. For example, some people need one aspirin

---

The Institute Formula is now available in health food stores and other retail outlets under various brand names. To ensure buying the Formula and not an imitation product, look for these ingredients on the label: "Specially prepared extracts of soya lecithin, providing phosphatidyl ethanolamine, phosphatidylcholine, phosphatidyl inositol; plant mucopolysaccharides derived from red seaweed and Irish moss (Chondrus crispus); niacin, 5.5 milligrams; and silicon dioxide."

to get rid of a headache, some need two or more, and others have bad reactions to aspirin and have to take a substitute pain reliever. (Fortunately, these are few, and the people who have shown allergic reactions to lecithin, choline or other ingredients of the Institute Formula are definitely a very tiny minority.)

The Institute Formula is available in powder, capsule and tablet form, but research has demonstrated that the tablet is most acceptable to most people. The average preventive dosage has been shown to be two tablets, two or three times a day, for a total dosage of approximately 4 grams a day. That is the saturation amount for the first thirty days, after which we recommend bringing it down to two tablets a day as a maintenance level for general conditions—that is, for people who have no symptoms of degenerative disease.

For people who are diseased or in really great danger of uncontrollable risk factors such as hereditary predisposition to heart disease, the tablets aren't enough. In such cases I recommend the powdered form of the Institute Formula. For those who have had heart attacks or strokes and are trying to rebuild their health, the optimum amount is 10 grams a day. Since each teaspoonful of the powder contains 4½ grams, these people should take a rounded tablespoonful each day.

The Rest of the Program

I have to emphasize that the Institute Formula is only one part of the Institute Program. If you take the formula as directed, but continue to eat a high-saturated-fat diet, sit around with little or no attempt at exercise, smoke cigarettes and drink excessive amounts of alcohol, you might as well try to cross the Atlantic Ocean in a rowboat. You may stay afloat for a while, but you won't reach your destination, which is a state of good health, free of degenerative diseases.

In the following chapters I will explain the importance of the other branches of the Institute Program and how they can help you to achieve your destination. And there's one extra ingredient that can't be measured by the spoonful but has an immeasurable effect on any self-improvement program: optimism.

Remember the story of the optimist and the pessimist who were each shown half a glass of water? The pessimist said it was half empty, but the optimist called it half full. The sincere belief that the Institute Program can make your life richer, more rewarding, more enjoyable and more fun can make your glass a lot more than half full. With spoonfuls of the Institute Formula added, I hope your cup "runneth over!"

Chapter 6

YOUR DIET—WHAT YOU EAT BECOMES YOU

It is literally true that many Americans are eating themselves to death—living to eat rather than eating to live.

I wrote these words in 1951 for an article in the *Journal of the American Medical Association* on the subject of arteriosclerosis. The article opened with a statement that made waves:

> *Until recently, arteriosclerosis was regarded as an incurable state—the inevitable result of advancing age and the remorseless effect of wear and tear or "rusting out" of the arteries.*
>
> *Accumulated evidence refutes these fatalistic resignations, stressing the concept that atherosclerosis is a metabolic error, in which disorders of the blood lipids and lipoproteins play a dominant role.*

As a result of statements like this—and the fact that my two teams of investigators were beginning to publish research to support them—I began to have an idea how Columbus must have felt when he first tried to tell people that the world was round. Of course, I wasn't the only person (or the only doctor) in the world who believed that lipid intake was related to arteriosclerosis and that diets in this country were destructive, but those of us who held these theories were considered to be crackpots. We were laughed at, and that was one of the milder forms of putdown we experienced in the 1940s and 1950s.

The very idea of introducing a diet that would change **119** the eating habits of the most powerful and affluent country in the world was an affront in the eyes of many. I had attacked one of the great American institutions, and I wasn't about to be let off with just a slap on the wrist.

After I tried to seriously promote my belief that Americans ate far too much fat and could improve their health by cutting down on such national favorites as bacon and eggs, steak, whipped cream and butter, the attacks began in earnest. My wife, Rita, and I spent many sleepless nights. My statements were condemned as being repugnant. I was threatened. It was proposed that I be expelled from some of the leading medical societies. The hospitals with which I was affiliated looked askance at me. My theories were so radical and frightening, and created such an emotional reaction, that many of my friends and colleagues were afraid to be seen with me!

Looking back over the past thirty-five years, I try to be a bit charitable. After all, the late 40s and early 50s were very reactionary times, and new ideas were looked upon with a great deal of suspicion. We had only recently survived World War II, and people were trying to get back to normal, not strike out in unheard-of new directions. Butter and sugar had been scarce to the point of rationing during the war, and people had suffered through "meatless Tuesdays" in efforts at conservation. And here I was telling them that all the delicious foods they were looking forward to being able to eat again were bad for them. I was before my time, and that can be a terrible experience.

Gradually, however, attitudes began to change. On the scientific level, other investigators began realizing the dangers of fatty diets, and connections between dietary fat and coronary disease were being confirmed in laboratories, animal studies and human clinical trials. In the early 60s, these theories gained acceptance by the Surgeon General's office and the public health services, and the tide started to turn. The public learned the words "cholesterol," "saturated" and "polyunsaturated." Obesity was recognized as being a factor in health as well as looks. And from being an object of attack, slowly but surely I became a curiosity.

Some of the incidents from that difficult time in the 50s were funny, now that I can look back on them without wincing. In restaurants, and at parties Rita and I attended, people who knew of my work would watch me, actually peer over my shoulder and take notes on what I had ordered and what I ate and drank.

Once, when Rita and I gave a party at our home in London, we were challenged by a guest who claimed to be the richest woman in the world. She had worked with Albert Schweitzer in the jungle for several years and was very eccentric and outspoken. She knew all about my work with diets and cholesterol and had followed my suggestions rigidly for some time.

The caterer had been unable to get some of the special foods we had ordered for the party, and at the last minute had substituted whatever was available. When the "richest woman" saw the waiters setting out cheeses, cold-cuts and even deviled eggs, she just couldn't hold her tongue. Regarding me with great disapproval, she mistakenly addressed me as "Professor" and sternly said, "Professor Morrison, how dare you talk so fervently about one thing and not practice what you preach."

I was completely taken aback. I could only explain with some embarrassment that Rita and I do practice what we preach, but that we do not feel in a position to dictate to others. Our friends may be less selective than we are and, after all (I said somewhat feebly), it is still a free country. I don't think I completely convinced her of my good intentions, but I was reminded again how careful one must be after becoming a preacher of any sort.

Now, of course, I feel completely vindicated. Even the American Heart Association—an organization that is not known for jumping on bandwagons or changing its mind in a hurry—acknowledges the proven connection between lipids and heart disease and promotes restriction of dietary fat.

In 1976, the *Journal of the American Medical Association* (the official publication of another group that is super-cautious and slow to accept change) published an article by Robert I. Levy, M.D., former director of the National Heart, Lung and Blood Institute, in which this noted physician wrote:

> *We now know that elevated lipid levels are the result of increased production or decreased removal of specific lipoproteins. . . . Treatment should always begin with an appropriate dietary prescription, which should be continued even after drug treatment is introduced, because the combined therapeutic effect is additive. Before administering a drug, the patient should be maintained on a diet for two to six weeks, at which time lipid values should be monitored regularly. If there is no alteration in baseline levels, therapy may be supplemented with a drug.*

In other words, the diet should come first, and drugs

should be added only if a patient is too seriously ill to be helped by dietary changes alone.

In January of 1981, an article appeared in the prestigious *New England Journal of Medicine* that confirmed my beliefs once and for all. (I didn't need to be convinced, of course—I had been convinced thirty-five years ago—but anyone who remains skeptical of the importance of a low-fat diet should read this article.) The authors were Richard B. Shekelle, Ph.D., and his associates in the now-famous Western Electric Study sponsored in part by the American Heart Association. They wrote:

> *Decreasing the proportion of calories obtained from saturated fatty acids, increasing the proportion from polyunsaturated fatty acids, and decreasing the amount of dietary cholesterol . . . will lower the average serum cholesterol in a group by predictable amounts.*

Their conclusion was that "lipid composition of the diet affects serum cholesterol concentration and risk of coronary death in middle-aged American men."

To cap it all, the famous nutrition researcher and epidemiologist, Jeremiah Stamler, M.D., of Northwestern University was quoted by *Time* magazine as having said in June of 1981, "If we could get more diet changes in the U.S. there would not be a big coronary problem in this country."

The temptation to say, "So there," is strong, but I'd rather say, "So here." Here is my dietary advice, based on many years of exhaustive scientific research, and included as part of the Institute Program to combat degenerative diseases.

The Basic Food Groups

There are three basic groups into which foods fall: Proteins, Fats and Carbohydrates. All are organic components of the foods we eat, and all are essential to our health. The key to good nutrition lies in balancing them.

Proteins

Proteins have been called "building blocks" because they are the basis of the formation and maintenance of all the body's tissues. In the body, they are converted into amino acids, which must constantly be replaced because the body has no way of storing them. Proteins also help to promote growth and regulate digestion, and they are essential to the formation of antibodies (infection fighters).

Since the body is continually building and rebuilding itself, protein is essential to life and good health. If you don't eat enough protein-rich foods, the lack will quickly become evident, first in such obvious problems as dull, listless hair, ridged nails, and weak muscles. If, on the other hand, you take in more protein than you need, the excess will be either used as energy or converted into fat.

How Much Protein Do You Need? Protein requirements vary according to age and sex. Children, whose bodies use protein for growth, need about 23 to 34 grams a day. Men, who are generally larger than women and have more body tissues to maintain, require about 45 to 56 grams each day, whereas women can get along with a bit less, approximately 44 to 46 grams per day. If a woman is pregnant or nursing, however, her needs are increased, since extra protein is needed for the growth of her baby or the production of milk. Pregnancy requires an additional 30 grams of protein per day, while nursing mothers should have about 20 grams a day more than usual.

Does that seem like a lot? It all depends on how you look at it. Most Americans take in approximately 100 grams of protein every day, which is almost twice as much as the highest requirement for an adult man. Since this protein is not all needed, the extra amount will be used for energy or converted to fat. And since we almost always get as much energy as we need (or more) from the other food forms, what's left? Right: fat. Add to that the fact that most of our protein comes from animal (saturated-fat) sources, and you can see that Americans are not only over-fatted but over-proteined as well.

Where Do We Get Our Protein? The bulk of dietary protein comes from animal sources: meat, fish, shellfish, poultry and dairy products (eggs, milk, cheese, cream, butter and yogurt). The rest is derived from specific plants: legumes (dried peas and beans, including soybeans), nuts (including nut products such as peanut butter) and wheat products (cereals, bread, flour and pasta).

Different foods contain different amounts of protein, and that's where selection becomes so important. For example, one serving of dried beans contains just as much protein as 2 ounces of cooked pork—but the beans will do you a lot more good and far less harm because they contain polyunsaturated vegetable fats rather than saturated animal fats.

Does all that mean you should give up meat and eat only beans? Not at all. But it does mean you should use common sense and applied knowledge in planning your meals; you can meet your protein requirements safely by eating more beans more often and less meat less often. It all comes back to balance.

Fats

I've already told you the basics about fats, but a review can only help you understand why controlling them is so important to your diet—and your life.

Fats supply energy (calories) in a concentrated form; they are needed for the maintenance of healthy, attractive (non-"dry") skin; and some also contribute the essential fatty acids (EFA). Some fats either provide or contribute to the absorption of vitamins A, D, E and K, which are appropriately called "fat-soluble vitamins."

When energy is needed, the body takes it from fats and carbohydrates first, leaving the protein to do its building job; for this reason, fats are said to be "protein-sparing." Finally, the EFAs are precursors—that is, essential steps in the manufacture—of hormonelike compounds called "prostaglandins," which are necessary for the proper function of blood platelets, the process of immunity and the contraction of smooth muscles.

Obviously, we cannot live without fats. And though the word "balance" may be getting a bit tiresome, we can't live without that, either. Too little fat would leave us without all the important functions mentioned in the previous paragraph—and too much fat both makes us unattractive and (far more important) contributes to heart disease.

Energy is measured in calories, and fats contain more calories than any other type of food. Whereas 1 ounce of a protein or carbohydrate food contains about 115 calories, 1 ounce of a fat food contains about 250 calories—more than twice the amount.

What Are the Types of Fat? As you know, fats are broken down into the categories of triglycerides, phospholipids and cholesterol.

To move through the body, lipids (another word for fats) join with protein molecules to become lipoproteins. The very-low-density lipoproteins (VLDL) and low-density lipoproteins

(LDL) deliver dangerous cholesterol to cells and contribute to the development of arteriosclerosis. The high-density lipoproteins (HDL) are able to *remove* dangerous cholesterol from cells and help to protect us against arteriosclerosis.

Fats are further classified as saturated and polyunsaturated. The saturated fats, which come mostly from animal sources, deliver high amounts of cholesterol, triglycerides, LDL and VLDL—they should be limited. The polyunsaturated fats, which come mostly from plant sources, deliver moderate amounts of necessary cholesterol and triglycerides, as well as high amounts of HDL—they should be used for most of your fat intake.

How can you tell the difference between saturated and polyunsaturated fats? In general, saturated fats are animal-derived, are solid at room temperature and are called fats; they include butter, lard and the fat on meat. On the other hand, most polyunsaturated fats are plant-derived, liquid at room temperature and are called oils; they include soybean oil, corn oil, safflower oil and so on—but *not* coconut oil. (In fact, coconut oil is 92 percent saturated fat and should be strictly avoided on a heart-disease-preventive diet, as should all products of the coconut.)

Today, package labeling is a big help to anyone who wants to control fat intake. Most "good" fat products—that is, those that are low in cholesterol and saturated fats—will bear "Nutritional Information" labels telling you how much fat the product contains and how much of that fat is polyunsaturated (P) and saturated (S). The general rule is that, to be good for a heart-disease-preventive diet, a fat product should contain at least twice as much polyunsaturated fat as saturated fat—this value is expressed as the "P/S ratio" and should be at least 2:1.

Interestingly, you will not find Nutritional Information labels on most "bad" fat products—those that are high in cholesterol and saturated fats. It makes sense from the manufacturers' point of view. They know their products are full of the ingredients health-conscious people want to avoid, so in the interest of selling more products, they don't advertise the fact. A good rule to follow is, If you don't see a Nutritional Information label, and don't already know what's in the product, don't buy it.

How Much Fat Do You Need? Fat requirements are different for children and adults, men and women. So are calorie requirements. And you are, above all, an individual with individual requirements in all areas. So I cannot give you a specific number and say, "This is how much fat *you* need every day." For that you will have to see your doctor, learn your actual weight and your ideal weight, and have your blood-lipid and lipoprotein levels measured.

In general, doctors who are aware of the dangers of fats as they relate to heart disease recommend that adults consume (1) no more than 300 milligrams of cholesterol each day (preferably less); (2) less than 10 percent of their total daily calories from saturated fats; and (3) about 10 percent of their total daily calories from polyunsaturated fats.

Whereas many doctors still believe that a P/S ratio of 1:1 is safe, I disagree, based on my many years of research in this field. My low-fat diet, and this branch of the Institute Program, are based on a P/S ratio of at least 2:1, and, if you follow the diet rigorously, 4:1.

Also, I think the levels of blood lipids in adults that most doctors consider acceptable are too high. My opinion is that the acceptable blood-lipid levels for adults are approximately:

Total cholesterol	135–250 milligrams (at age 40)*
Total triglycerides	30–135 milligrams
VLDL	0–40 milligrams
LDL	62–185 milligrams
HDL	29–77 milligrams

(*For coronary-risk patients, total cholesterol should not exceed 220 milligrams.)

Remember that the only way you can find out what your blood-lipid levels are is to have the appropriate tests performed by your doctor. Be sure to specify that you want the VLDL, LDL and HDL fractions done—otherwise you'll only get total cholesterol, and we now know that that's not enough information.

Where Do We Get Our Fats? The obvious sources are plain to see—fat rings meat and occurs inside it as "marbling." Fat occurs in solid form as butter, lard and shortening, and in liquid form as salad oil or cooking oil.

There are also numerous hidden sources of fat—you can't see it, but it is plentiful in milk, cheese, cream, chocolate, nuts, corn, avocadoes and coconuts. To separate these into the saturated and polyunsaturated categories, consider the source: Meat, milk, butter, cheese and lard come from animals and contain primarily saturated fats; nuts, corn, cocoa beans (chocolate) and avocadoes, being plants, contain primarily polyunsaturated fats. You already know about the coconuts.

Carbohydrates

These food components, which are made up of carbon, hydrogen and oxygen, come in two forms: starches and sugars. They supply us with energy and influence the levels of glucose (sugar) in our blood. Like fats, they are "protein-sparing"— that is, they will be called upon first when the body needs energy, leaving the protein to do its work of building and repairing tissues. Most carbohydrates contribute fiber, vitamins and minerals to the body, as well as help in the metabolic processes that put these nutrients to good use.

Carbohydrates are divided between the digestible parts and the "indigestible" parts called "fiber." The term "indigestible" is a bit misleading, however. It does not mean that you can't eat the fiber (on the contrary, it is recommended) or that doing so will give you indigestion. It does mean that the fiber content of foods (which is generally found in plant cell walls) is not absorbed into the bloodstream in the form of nutrients. Instead, it passes undigested into the intestine, where it absorbs water and aids in the process of elimination.

Recent research has stressed the importance of substantial amounts of fiber or food bulk in the diet because of its value in providing protection against malignant growths in the intestinal tract. This can be provided by balanced supplies of vegetables, fruits and greens, as described in this chapter.

What about the Sugars? We all know that sugar is high in calories and that it is "bad for the teeth," promoting cavities. It's also true that some people (diabetics) cannot metabolize sugar properly and are in danger if they do not control their sugar intake very carefully. It is *not* true that eating too much sugar will give you diabetes; however, eating too much sugar will add to your weight, provide very little in the way of nutrition, and promote cavities in your teeth.

On the other hand, a certain amount of sugar is necessary for life, and the answer again is balance. Like fats, sugars come in various forms; some occur naturally in vegetables and fruits (especially fruits, which is why they taste sweet), while others occur naturally in honey, molasses and sugar cane. The best kinds are the natural kinds. The trouble-causing sugars are the refined and processed kinds—the white sugar most people love to put in their coffee and tea, not to mention the "unseen" sugar that exists in great quantities in candy, cake, cookies, ice cream, chocolate sauce, canned fruits and drinks, both soft and hard (alcoholic).

Most adults in the United States today get about 46 percent of their energy supply from carbohydrates—22 percent from starches and 24 percent from sugars. When we break down the 24 percent we get from sugars, we find that 6 percent of our energy comes from natural sugars and 18 percent from refined and processed sugars.

Is that too much? Yes. Refined and processed sugars are unknown in nature and were never part of nature's plan for human nutrition. They were created by man for their sweet taste, and that plus calories is about all they provide. By reducing the amount of refined sugar you eat, you will be helping to keep your weight down to a healthy level and your teeth less susceptible to cavities. Natural sugars can be just as satisfying to your taste, as you'll learn once you get used to them.

How Much Carbohydrate Do You Need? On the average, most adults should have a minimum of 50 to 100 grams of digestible carbohydrate each day, an amount that is easy to get from nutritious cereals, vegetables and whole wheat bread. You can, for example, get about 26 grams of digestible carbohydrate from two slices of whole wheat bread, 28 grams from one cup of bran flakes (without sugar), and 25 grams from half a cup of brown or enriched rice. That's 79 grams right there. Add half a cup of cooked peas (10 grams) and one fresh orange (16 grams), and you have 105 grams of digestible carbohydrate, along with a lot of valuable nutrients.

How much carbohydrate is too much? Again, that depends on your age, your weight, your sex and the amount of physical exercise you get. It also depends on the type of carbohydrate you eat. If you add 2 tablespoons of refined sugar (22 grams of digestible carbohydrate) to the cup of bran flakes mentioned in the last paragraph, then drink an 8-ounce glass of soda (about 33 grams) and treat yourself to a dessert of 2 ounces of chocolate candy (28 grams), you will have taken in another 83 grams of carbohydrate and have practically nothing to show for it but a lot of excess calories that will have to be worked off—and your dentist may profit from your indulgence, to boot.

However, don't be discouraged and think that you have to give up sweets altogether. Once you have determined which of my low-fat diets is best for you as an individual, you'll see that there is plenty of provision for pampering your sweet tooth—*without* making it decay or adding obesity and arteriosclerosis to your health profile.

Where Do We Get Our Carbohydrates? The starch forms of carbohydrates occur naturally in wheat and wheat products as well as in vegetables such as corn, potatoes, rice and legumes (peas and beans). Human ingenuity has invented plenty of forms of starch foods that we eat regularly: flour, bread, cereal, spaghetti, noodles, macaroni, dumplings, pastry and so on.

The sugar forms, which occur naturally in honey, molasses, syrups, sugar cane, fruits and some vegetables, have been processed and hidden in a myriad of delicious but almost worthless man-made products, as mentioned earlier in this section: candy, cake, cookies, ice cream, chocolate sauce, canned fruits, soda pop and liquor.

What Are Calories —and How Much Do They Count?

Calories are units of energy, and they are very important. Everything you swallow (with the exception of water, of course) is going to contribute calories.

On the other hand, everything you do (even sleeping and breathing) is going to use up calories. The more active you are, the more calories you will use up. The less active you are, the fewer calories you will use up—and those that are not used will stay in your body as fat.

The amount of calories you need is a matter of (you guessed it) balancing the amount you take in against the amount you use up. This is only one reason why you should see your doctor before you choose and begin a diet. Maybe you need to lose weight—that means fewer calories and more activity. Perhaps your weight is right for your age, sex, height and bone structure—that means changing the quality (very few saturated fats and more polyunsaturates) rather than the quantity of calories to guard against degenerative diseases. Or you may even be underweight—that means both improving the quality and increasing the quantity of your calories, as well as regulating your activities to provide healthy exercise that will use up the *right* number of calories instead of too many.

Your diet will have to be tailored for you, not for the average man or woman, because the "average" man or woman is an imaginary being made up of statistics, not a real person.

Foods: The Right and the Wrong

Arteriosclerosis is as deadly a weapon as a gun—it just takes a lot longer to kill you. It is diet—the wrong diet—that helps to cock the trigger of this weapon that is aimed point-blank at your heart. Whether or not that trigger is ever pulled will depend, admittedly, on a number of other factors as well as diet: heredity, the occurrence of other diseases, hormones, stress, biochemical factors and so on. But why play Russian roulette with your heart?

By eliminating the wrong foods from your diet, by including the right foods in the right amounts, and by using the Institute Formula, you can achieve up to an 81 percent protection (as estimated by statisticians) against the degenerative diseases that lead to arteriosclerosis, heart attack and stroke.

But what are the right and the wrong foods? That's not a simple question to answer. A proper diet is the easiest and safest "medicine" a doctor can prescribe. Yet doctors have found diets to be the most difficult prescriptions for their patients to follow. Most people are so firmly established in their eating patterns, and so discouraged by the fact that the results of a good diet are slow to come and hard to see, that they don't stay with their prescribed diets for very long. They follow a stop-and-go routine that provides little benefit.

"Diet" is, unfortunately, a negative word. If you play a word-association game with people and ask them what comes to mind when you say "diet," the answers will be "deprivation," "frustration," "hunger," "will-power," "won't power," "craving" or "forbiddance." But that attitude is, again, like the pessimist looking at the half glass of water. Diets, believe it or not, can be delicious. They can be satisfying, never subjecting you to that "half-empty" feeling that makes you crave something you shouldn't have. They can be varied and interesting—in fact, doctors know that a boring diet is a born failure because many people simply cannot stick to it. As soon as their boredom becomes intolerable, they'll either drop their diet completely or go off on a temporary "food binge," stuffing themselves with all the wrong foods, then falling into an awful feeling of guilt. So a diet has to keep you happy in order to keep you healthy—and that's the goal I've aimed for in constructing my low-fat diet (a type of diet, by the way, that was *originated* by our Institute).

Some people are allergic or sensitive to certain foods. They may know, for example, that if they eat strawberries, they'll break out in a rash. Like an allergic person, you now know that if you eat too much saturated fat, you may break out in a rash of arteriosclerotic plaques—and they're all the more dangerous because you can't see them. If you think of yourself as being truly allergic to saturated fat and cholesterol, it won't be so hard to avoid the foods that contain them. Pretty soon you won't even miss them.

	The Right Foods	**The Wrong Foods**
Appetizers	Fresh vegetables Cheese (low-fat) and crackers Low-fat canapes Peanuts Unbuttered popcorn Marinated herring Stuffed egg whites	Caviar Fatty cheeses Creamed dips Stuffed pastry puffs Creamed shellfish Buttered popcorn Creamed herring Deviled eggs
Salads	Almost anything	Dressings made with cream or mayonnaise
Soups	Bouillon Vegetable broth Defatted soups	Creamed soups Fatty chowders
Meats	Very lean beef (broiled) White veal (broiled) Chicken (white meat) Turkey (white meat)	Bacon Ham Pork Duck Goose Brains and sweetbreads Sausages Liver
Fish	Sole Sea bass Flounder Red snapper Perch Haddock Sturgeon Smelts Water-packed tuna	Brook trout Porgy Cod Oil-packed tuna
Dairy Products	Skim milk Low-fat cheese Low-fat yogurt Egg whites Egg substitutes Margarine	Whole milk Fatty cheese Whole milk yogurt Egg yolks Whole eggs Butter
Vegetables	Raw or steamed vegetables	Creamed, buttered or fried vegetables
Fruits	Almost anything	Coconut
Desserts	Fresh fruit Ice milk (low-fat) Frozen yogurt (low-fat) Angel food cake Sherbet Gelatin	Coconut Ice cream Pastry made with butter Egg custard Whipped cream Pudding

A heartening fact is that for almost every wrong food, there is a right food that can be substituted. Today, technology has provided us with some modifications of wrong foods that taste just as good or better than the originals—for example, defatted milk and egg substitutes. So don't think of the low-fat, low-cholesterol diet as a deprivation. Instead, think of it as a gift—a gift of nature and knowledge that is a lifelong plan for a longer, healthier life.

Here is a very basic list of the right and wrong foods for a healthy, tasty, satisfying and effective low-fat, low-cholesterol diet. I'll tell you more about each category later—this is just a list that you can copy, frame and hang in your kitchen as a reminder.

There are two very important things to remember about this list. First, as I have pointed out, it is a *basic* list, covering only general categories of food. Second, it is a list of low-saturated-fat foods, not of low-calorie foods.

Because individuals have different needs, there are very few health recommendations that can be applied to everybody. Nevertheless, I can state flatly that I believe *everybody* should follow a low-saturated-fat diet, one that virtually eliminates the dangerous fats that carry LDL and VLDL cholesterol but supplies the necessary polyunsaturated fats and their protective HDL cholesterol.

Calories are another matter. Even among people with normal or low blood-lipid levels, calorie requirements are very different depending on age, sex, activity and bone structure. A low-calorie diet is not right for everyone.

How many calories do *you* need each day? Again, there are very basic guidelines, calculated by scientists for people of "average" activity and bone structure and normal weight. The accompanying table will tell you *approximately* how many calories you need each day, assuming that your weight is normal. (See weight table in chapter 3.)

You can see at a glance that children of both sexes have the same basic calorie requirements. But from the teens on, boys and men need more calories than girls and women. Why? Because, in general, males are bigger than females, are more physically active and have higher rates of metabolism. (There are exceptions, of course—a male office worker, for instance, is far less physically active than a female ballerina.)

Calorie requirements have their steepest drop for both sexes after age 50 because both metabolism and physical activity slow down as we move through middle age toward senior citizenry. That's a tough time—by middle age our eating pat-

DAILY CALORIE REQUIREMENTS

AGE (years)	WEIGHT (pounds)	HEIGHT (inches)	MALE	FEMALE
1 to 3	29	35	1,300	1,300
4 to 6	44	44	1,700	1,700
7 to 10	62	52	2,400	2,400
11 to 14	99	62	2,700	
11 to 14	101	62		2,200
15 to 18	145	69	2,800	
15 to 18	120	64		2,100
19 to 22	154	70	2,900	
19 to 22	120	64		2,100
23 to 50	154	70	2,700	
23 to 50	120	64		2,000
51 to 75	154	70	2,400	
51 to 75	120	64		1,800
76 and over	154	70	2,050	
76 and over	120	64		1,600

SOURCE: Adapted from *Recommended Dietary Allowances*, 9th ed., by the Committee on Dietary Allowances (Washington, D.C.: National Research Council, National Academy of Sciences, 1980).

terns are pretty solidly set, and it's not easy to start eating less just because the calendar is getting harder to look at. It's the reason so many middle-aged and elderly people are overweight. But it doesn't have to happen. If you can form good eating habits in your youth or young adulthood, you'll find that awareness of the subtle changes taking place in your body will be a strong incentive toward reducing your calorie intake or maintaining physical activity into your later years.

To repeat, these figures are general. The only way you can be sure of your own, personal calorie requirement is to see your doctor for a checkup.

Now let's take a closer look at the categories of right and wrong foods and get a little more specific about what you can safely eat and what you should strictly avoid.

Appetizers

Most of us don't encounter appetizers unless we are eating out or are either the guests or the hosts at a party. But there's no reason to cheat on your diet and harm your body just because the occasion is special.

Most appetizers, of course, are concoctions rather than single ingredients. But think of the good things you can choose if you're reading a menu or wandering around a party peering at the plates of tempting hors d'oeuvres the host has set out.

A relish tray is excellent. It usually holds raw celery, carrots, radishes, cucumber sticks, green peppers and little cherry tomatoes, all of which are both delicious and free of saturated fat. The problem comes when you pick up one of those good nibbles and your eye falls on the dip.

What's in the dip? Usually trouble; dips are often made with sour cream, cream cheese, cheddar cheese, bleu cheese—all dangerously high in saturated fat. However, many hosts nowadays are aware of these dangers (and if you are the host or hostess, you can of course control this yourself) and provide dips made with low-fat yogurt or low-fat cottage cheese. Yogurt has become so popular lately that you can buy it in any supermarket, and the low-fat brands are clearly labeled "low fat." Dips made with this dairy product (which tastes very much like sour cream) are every bit as delicious as those made with saturated-fat products. You can add herbs, spices, ketchup, curry powder, almost anything your imagination comes up with, and have a dip people will rave about.

You can also find low-fat, low-cholesterol cheeses in supermarkets, and your guests aren't likely to know the difference. If you are the guest, you won't know what kind of cheese is being served, so it's best to skip the cheese if you must keep your saturated-fat intake low. (For an individual whose blood-lipid level is low or normal, and whose uncontrollable risk factors are favorable, an occasional high-fat cheese is acceptable, but even such a person must remember the word "occasional" if he goes to a lot of parties.)

Canapes can be made of almost anything, so you have to be choosy. Mushrooms on toast, for example, are fine—as long as they haven't been broiled in butter. Caviar on crackers with chopped egg yolks is best left on the tray; both caviar and egg yolks are extremely high in dangerous cholesterol. Anything containing shrimp, crab meat or lobster has to be labeled "limited," since shellfish are known to be high in cholesterol, but not as dangerously high as many other foods. (The jury is still out on the protective HDL cholesterol content of shellfish.)

Stay away from creamed mixtures served in puff pastry.

Unless the baker is conscious of saturated fat and cholesterol, the puff pastry will have been made with an unconscionable amount of butter, and the sauce with heavy cream. On the other hand, if you are giving a party and want to serve hot hors d'oeuvres of that nature, you can make your own puff pastry with polyunsaturated margarine and your "cream" sauce with low-fat milk. There are so many delicious alternatives to the tasty bad habits we've acquired!

Deviled eggs, for example, are traditionally made by mixing the yolk of the egg with other flavorings and stuffing them inside the hard-boiled egg white. If you are the cook, hard boil the eggs, get rid of the yolks and stuff the whites with a low-saturated-fat filling. Your guests will probably ask, "What's *in* these great stuffed eggs?" and think of you as a truly innovative cook.

If you like herring as an appetizer, you've no doubt seen that it comes packed in jars, either marinated or creamed. Stick to the marinated herring—it's just as flavorful and pays off in health benefits.

Popcorn and peanuts are another matter. Plain popcorn is fine, but not many people like their popcorn plain. If you must "butter" it, use polyunsaturated margarine instead of butter—but remember (if you must limit your calories) that margarine and butter contain exactly the same number of calories, about 100 per teaspoonful. Peanuts contain acceptable polyunsaturated peanut oil (though their P/S ratio is only 1:1)—but they are both habit-forming and fattening, so you have to let your knowledge of your own calorie requirements act as your conscience. Excellent substitutes are roasted soybeans, sunflower seeds and pumpkin seeds.

Commercial products such as cheese puffs and potato chips should be avoided—unless you can be sure the potato chips have been fried in polyunsaturated oil and your weight is low or normal. Cheese puffs are not recommended in any case.

Salads

The list of ingredients with which you can make a salad is almost endless and almost universally good. Lettuce, tomatoes, cucumbers, carrots, green pepper, onions, mushrooms and so on are all good. What you have to watch out for is the dressing.

Oil-and-vinegar salad dressings are good if you don't have to limit calories, and *very* good if they're made with soybean or safflower oil (high in polyunsaturated fat). But creamy dressings are made with heavy cream, and mayonnaise is made with egg yolks.

A chef's salad made with ham and cheese is best avoided. Chicken salad made with white meat and a mayonnaise substitute is fine. Tuna salad (again made with a mayonnaise substitute) is good for low-calorie dieters if the tuna is packed in water. Egg salad can be just as good made without the yolks and with a mayonnaise substitute.

Soups

What could be better than a hearty dish of hot soup on a cold day? A hearty dish of hot *low-fat* soup.

Creamed soups are dangerous foods. If you're a cook, you know that many recipes for creamed soup even tell you to add a lump of butter to keep the soup from puckering! The saturated-fat content is frightening.

You can, however, make your own "creamed" soups with low-fat milk, enriched with low-fat milk powder. Even clam chowder can be made this way.

Onion soup is usually topped off with a generous dollop of grated cheese—use a low-fat cheese like parmesan, and you can have the same delectable taste without the saturated fat.

Vegetable soups are all excellent for a low-fat diet—but many of them are made with meat-stock broths that are high in invisible saturated fat. If you make your own, you can get rid of the fat and retain the flavor and protein (see the section on cooking methods later in this chapter). If you buy canned soup, put the can in the refrigerator for about an hour before you open it. You'll be amazed at the clumps of congealed fat you'll see floating on the surface after a good chilling. Toss them out, and the soup is safe to eat.

Meats

To enjoy a low-saturated-fat diet, you don't have to give up meat unless you want to. You just have to be a choosy and careful cook.

Lean beef and veal are acceptable on my special diet, but I recommend that you eat them once in a while instead of several times a week. When you do eat them, select the leanest cuts you can find, and cut off as much of the visible fat as possible. Then broil and drain (for the how-to of this technique, see the section on cooking methods later in this chapter).

The white meat of chicken and turkey is much lower in fat than the dark meat. These meats should be eaten without the skin, since that is where these birds deposit most of their fat.

Meats to avoid because of calories as well as cholesterol are pork (including ham and bacon), organ meats such as liver, brains, kidneys and sweetbreads, sausages (which are usually made with pork and tremendous amounts of fat) and duck and goose, the fattiest birds in the air.

If you like gravy with your meat, don't despair. Gravy does not have to be made with the pan drippings from the meat you've cooked—those drippings are largely pure, saturated animal fat. You can separate the fat, keep the flavorful juices, and make a fat-free gravy (see instructions in the cooking methods section later in this chapter).

Fish

Most fish are very low in fat and are also excellent sources of protein. Those listed under "Right Foods" are especially low, while those under "Wrong Foods" are somewhat higher—but not as high as the meats in the same column. Almost any fish is a good meal unless you are strictly watching your calorie intake.

Caviar is an exception, being very high in dangerous cholesterol. Since it is also extremely expensive, it shouldn't be too difficult to sacrifice.

A puzzling fish is the salmon. Researchers tell us that when the salmon is swimming upstream on its perilous journey to the spawning ground, it is very high in fat. After it has exhausted its energies and is floating lazily back downstream, however, its fat content is very low. But it isn't likely that the person who sells you the salmon will know which way it was swimming when it was caught. Unless your diet must be severely restricted, enjoy a salmon once in a while—but please skip the mayonnaise or hollandaise sauce.

Shellfish (shrimp, crab, lobster, clams, oysters, mussels and so on) once were thought to be dangerously high in both fat and cholesterol. However, recent reports by food chemists suggest that there is only a modest elevation in cholesterol content, balanced by a considerable elevation in polyunsaturated essential fatty acids. Shellfish are still higher in fat than shell-less fish, however, and should be kept on your "once-in-a-while" list unless you are very lean and blessed with a low-to-normal blood-lipid level.

Dairy Products

If you're old enough to remember the days when milk was delivered to your door in bottles, you probably remember that there was an inch or two of heavy, thick liquid at the top of the bottle that was pure cream. That's where the fat and cholesterol collected (fat is lighter than water and therefore floats to the top). To get whole milk, you had to shake the bottle to mix the two together, and many people kept them separate, using the cream for whipping or pouring into coffee or on cereal.

Nowadays, when you have to go to the supermarket to buy milk in waxed paper cartons (unless you live on a farm), the mixing has already been done, and the milk stays mixed—that's why it says "homogenized" right on the carton.

Skim milk, on the other hand, is what you got in the old days if you did not mix the contents of the bottle; the cream is skimmed off the top and sold separately, and the "bottom part" remains rich in protein and vitamin D, but free of the butterfat and cholesterol that can fatten you and promote the formation of arteriosclerotic plaques.

You need the nutrients in skim milk and should have at least one pint a day, whether you drink it straight or mix it with other foods. If you miss the rich, creamy taste of whole milk, try mixing in one or more tablespoonsful of dried, low-fat milk powder. This powder not only adds richness and taste but is extremely high in protein and vitamins. Its uses are many and valuable; you can add it to sauces and gravies to thicken them and give the illusion of the usual fatty, harmful mixes, or you can add it to low-fat cheese in making a dip, and you'll swear you're eating everyday, fatty cheese dip.

Cottage cheese has always had the reputation of being a solid fixture in weight-loss diets—but watch your step. It comes in two varieties, creamed and low-fat. The low-fat version says on the package "less than 4 percent butterfat," and this is what you should use. It's best not to order cottage cheese when eating in a restaurant, since chances are you'll be getting the creamed variety.

Cheese, as mentioned earlier, is also being defatted these days, so you need to do some label reading before buying. Look for the words "low-fat" and "low-chol." There are also some cheeses that are naturally low in butterfat and cholesterol, notably ricotta and mozzarella—that means you can still enjoy lasagna as long as you don't have to stay away from the pasta for your weight's sake. Mozzarella even comes in two varieties, whole-milk and part-skim-milk; the part-skim-milk is for you.

Cream cheese is out, but you can make a reasonable substitute by mixing low-fat milk powder with low-fat cottage cheese.

Yogurt is another dieter's delight, available in both whole and low-fat versions. It is perfect as a substitute for sour cream, except that it will curdle if cooked for more than a few minutes. But that's easily remedied—just wait until the last minute to add it to a hot sauce in place of sour cream, heat very gently while stirring it in, and you have the perfect sour-cream-sauce substitute.

Today yogurt is available in almost every supermarket, both plain and with fruit. The fruited varieties make delicious desserts, but if you're trying to lose weight, check the labels to see how much sugar they contain, and limit your use of them according to your dietary allowance.

Egg yolks are one of the richest sources of dangerous cholesterol available. I believe the time-honored custom of eating two eggs fried in bacon fat every morning contributes to the frightening rates of arteriosclerosis that now exist among our middle-aged and elderly populations—people who were fed that delicious-but-deadly breakfast all during their childhoods.

Here's where it pays to know your family history and your blood-lipid level. If there is little or no circulatory disease in your family tree, and your blood-lipid level is low, it's safe to eat one or two eggs a week—but please don't fry them in bacon fat; that's just tempting fate. If you must fry them, use polyunsaturated margarine; however, remember that margarine is high in calories and not recommended for the overweight.

Eggs also sneak into our diet in ways we might not suspect. If you cook, you know that eggs are used as a binding medium to hold meat loaves and meatballs together. They are mixed into pancakes, cakes, noodles, dumplings and some sauces. But you need not give up these foods because they are made with eggs; science has provided us with undetectable egg substitutes.

The egg substitutes now on the market can be found in the frozen-food section of your supermarket. They are specifically designed to give you the taste and texture of eggs without the dangerous cholesterol.

Cartons of egg substitute usually contain the equivalent of two whole eggs. You have to thaw them before use, then use them within a week after thawing. You can do everything with these substitutes that you can do with real eggs, with one exception—since they are in liquid form, you can't fry them and get the "sunny-side-up" appearance of an egg yolk surrounded by its white. But you can scramble them, and they can be used in cooking exactly as you would use real eggs. I recommend them highly.

You can even use egg substitutes to make your own noodles and other pastas if you're an ambitious cook. If not, use pastas sparingly, keeping your blood-lipid level in mind and remembering that they are made with real eggs as well as being high in calories.

Butter is another very rich source of saturated fat and dangerous cholesterol. But modern food technology has made it possible to create polyunsaturated margarine that tastes just like butter. You can spread it on toast, use it in sauces, and fry with it. But it bears repeating that margarine's calorie content is exactly the same as that of butter—keep that in mind if you have to limit your calories.

Vegetables

Vegetables are virtually fat-free and contain no cholesterol. That is one reason some people become vegetarians— but vegetarians have to be very careful to be sure they get enough of the protein they miss by not eating meat. You don't have to become a vegetarian in order to keep your lipid intake within healthy limits; however, it is a good idea to plan your meals to include lots of vegetables, especially raw ones.

Cooking can destroy the nutritional value of vegetables, but it doesn't have to. See the section of this chapter on cooking methods for safe and tasty ways of preparing these valuable foods.

Fruits

Like vegetables, fruits are entirely free of cholesterol and almost entirely free of fat, with two exceptions. As I have already told you, the coconut is one of the highest sources of dangerous cholesterol known to man. This includes coconut meat, milk, oil and the flaked coconut you often see on cakes and in the popular "snowball" dessert.

Like eggs, coconut can sneak into your diet. It is often mixed into cookies and candy (where you can usually spot it by taste), and it is completely hidden in such seemingly innocent foods as nondairy creamers and nondairy whipped toppings. In some of these products it is coconut oil that provides richness and thickness. You're much better off using skim milk for coffee and whipped egg whites (with a little sweetener added) as a dessert topping.

The avocado, while it is free of cholesterol, is nonetheless fattening, which you have to take into account if you are trying to lose weight.

Other than that, fruits are rich in nutrients and, because they contain the natural sugar fructose, can satisfy the sweet tooth as desserts. If you buy canned or frozen fruits, choose the "unsweetened" variety, which means that they are packed in their natural juices and no refined sugar or syrup has been added.

Desserts

Fresh fruit is the ideal dessert, but our sophisticated appetites want something a little different from time to time.

Do you have to give up ice cream to be safe? Technically yes, but there are substitutes that are just as satisfying. Ice cream is what its name implies—*cream* that has been iced, with sugar and flavoring added. But you can also get ice milk, which has less fat and, best of all, frozen low-fat yogurt, which is now available in almost every flavor man has ever devised for ice cream. Check the calorie content on the label, and limit your intake according to your needs, but don't feel deprived if you're an ice cream lover!

Commercially made cakes (except angel food, which is made with egg whites) contain both whole eggs and butter, and pie crust is made with butter, sometimes glazed with egg before baking. You can save your arteries and still have these desserts if you make your own, using egg substitutes and polyunsaturated margarine. You will, of course, have to keep their calories in mind if you're trying to lose weight.

Sherbet and gelatin desserts are made without fats, but the commercial brands may contain high amounts of refined sugar and thus be very fattening. Check the labels. If you are following a weight-loss diet, look for the dietetic brands of both these desserts. Custards and puddings, usually made with eggs and lots of refined sugar, are also available in cholesterol-free, artificially sweetened varieties.

What about chocolate? If there's anyone who doesn't like chocolate, I haven't met him, and frankly, I doubt that he exists. But the fat problem with chocolate originates with an ingredient that is used in commercial processing: whole milk (used in milk chocolate, not sweet or semi-sweet chocolate). The actual source of the chocolate flavor, the cocoa bean, is low in fat!

As far as I know, no one has yet devised a commercial chocolate product that is cholesterol-free. But you can make your own chocolate cake, frosting, brownies, puddings, sauce, and even syrup to pour over your frozen yogurt, just by substituting unsweetened cocoa for chocolate, polyunsaturated oil for butter or shortening (and, of course, a natural sweetener such as honey, molasses, date sugar, fructose or barley malt, for sugar). If you're not already a cook, you may become one to save your health and find that cooking is a lot of fun, an outlet for creative energy, and practical as well.

Cereals

There are no "wrong" cereals except for the commercial brands coated with refined sugar that add empty calories and attack your teeth. By now you also know better than to drown your cereal in cream or plop a pat of real butter on top of the hot varieties.

Cereals are nutritious, energy-producing and virtually saturated-fat-free. Therefore, all cooked or dry cereals are excellent carbohydrate foods, especially when served with skim milk, fruit, wheat germ and the powdered form of the Institute Formula. This combination will promote energy and increase endurance, thus lessening the degree to which you feel fatigue, and it includes a good measure of vitamins and minerals as a bonus. The taste of any cereal, as you probably already know, is enormously enhanced by the addition of fresh or stewed fruits—bananas, prunes, peaches, pears, apricots, berries, dates, figs, raisins, apples—the list is endless.

Whole wheat cereals and whole grain cereals are also an important source of vitamin B complex, protein and fiber in the low-fat diet. You can't go wrong with cereals, as long as you moisten them with skim milk and use a small amount of a natural sweetener.

Breads

Both white and whole wheat breads contain a negligible amount of fat (about 4 percent by weight), and a fairly small amount of protein (about 10 percent); the rest is carbohydrate.

Whole wheat bread is the most nutritious form of this food that has been called the "staff of life." White bread, stripped of the nutrient-rich germ and the fiber-rich bran, is more of a crutch than a staff.

Unfortunately, most commercial bakers make bread—that includes rolls, muffins, buns and coffee cake—with lard, butter and egg yolks. An exception is French bread, which is usually made without eggs.

However, bread is the only bakery product with which the French have been that restrained—French pastries are rich in eggs, and the delectable, flaky croissant is not only made with eggs and butter (lots of it!) but also brushed with egg before being put in the oven.

If you enjoy being a cook, it's a simple step to enjoy being a baker as well, making your own breads and pastries with egg substitutes and polyunsaturated margarine. Does anything equal the mouth-watering aroma of fresh bread in the oven?

If you're not a cook or baker, I suggest you stick to whole wheat and French bread—and use polyunsaturated margarine instead of butter as a spread.

Drinks

With the exception of milk, egg nog, hot chocolate, and the popular but dangerous piña colada, most drinks are free of saturated fat. They may, however, be very high in calories.

Your best bets are skim milk, fresh fruit juice and herb teas. Coffee and tea, while almost completely free of calories until cream, milk and sugar are added, nonetheless contain a lot of caffeine, which should be limited. (I'll tell you why in chapter 8.) Carbonated sodas are free of fat but very heavy in refined sugar—dentists have been speaking out against sugary sodas for as long as I can remember.

There are, of course, sugar-free varieties of most sodas. However, almost all of these are sweetened with saccharine, which has gotten some very bad press lately. I believe the best soft drinks are fresh, unsweetened fruit juices.

What about alcoholic drinks? Those made with cream (bacardis, grasshoppers and so on) and with coconut (piña colada) are very high in saturated fat and should be avoided.

Alcohol itself contains no fat, but is extremely high in sugar content. If you do not need to lose weight, and have no trouble limiting yourself to a couple of drinks, alcoholic beverages are not harmful—and wine can even be good for you in small amounts, as described in chapter 8.

The Way You Cook

Cooking methods can make a world of difference in both the fat content and calorie content of food—as well as either destroying or preserving the nutrients. Here are a few important guidelines for the cooks among my readers.

Frying

Frying adds calories. It also adds saturated fat and dangerous cholesterol if you fry with butter, lard or another animal-based fat.

If you and the people for whom you cook can afford the calories, it is preferable to fry lightly with polyunsaturated fats—that is, polyunsaturated margarine and the vegetable oils made from soybeans, safflowers and corn. But don't let frying get out of hand. Remember that the food you fry absorbs the fat and is much higher in calories than food cooked by other methods. Also, deep frying actually turns polyunsaturated fat into saturated fat.

Broiling

This method is designed to drain the fat off meats, while subjecting the outer surface to direct flame, producing a crisp crust that many people love. When you prepare beef, lamb chops or any other fatty meat, broiling is the preferred method—and you can lower the saturated-fat content even more by carefully trimming off as much visible fat as possible before putting the meat in the broiler.

Roasting

This method subjects your meat to dry heat but not a direct flame. If the meat is placed on a rack in the roasting pan, the fat will drip off and collect in the bottom of the pan, along with the juices. You can then perform the great Fat-Free Trick to get rid of the fat while preserving the juices for sauce or gravy.

The Fat-Free Trick. After the meat is done, set it aside and refrigerate the remaining contents of the roasting pan. The fat will float to the top, where the cool temperature of the refrigerator will cause it to solidify (remember, saturated fats are solid at room temperature, and the refrigerator just hastens the process). Then you can scrape the fat off, throw it away and have the delicious juices remaining in the bottom of the pan. The meat can be reheated if you plan to serve it hot.

The Fat-Free Trick can also be performed with soup stock made from meat or poultry. Make the stock ahead of time, then refrigerate it until the fat is solid. Scrape off and discard the fat, reheat the soup, and you'll have fat-free soup with all the taste and nutrients of the meat or poultry from which it was made.

If you can't take the time to refrigerate your pan drippings or soup, there is a gadget now available in the housewares sections of department stores (and in many mail-order catalogs) that does a good job of separating the fat for you. It is a plastic pitcher on which the spout is connected to the *bottom* of the bowl rather than the middle or top, as in ordinary pitchers. It operates on the principle that fat, being lighter than water, floats to the top. When you pour, the juices come out of the bottom of the pitcher, while the fat remains on top, trapped in the bowl of the pitcher. When the fat gets to the bottom, you just stop pouring and throw the fat away. One of these pitchers is an invaluable addition to your kitchen equipment.

You can also use the old-fashioned method of skimming the fat off the top of a soup pot or roasting pan with a pastry brush or paper towel, but that is time-consuming, messy and incomplete. The newer methods just described are preferable.

Boiling

Food should be boiled only if you plan to use the water in which it is boiled as part of the recipe. The reason is that during the boiling, vitamins and nutrients move out of the food and into the water.

Spinach provides a perfect example of this. If you boil spinach in water, when you are done you will have limp spinach and green water, and in that water are most of the vitamins and minerals. If you throw the water away, you'll be depriving yourself of most of the nutritive value of the vegetable.

Soup is another good example. When you make chicken soup, you boil the chicken and some vegetables in water. When you're done, both the flavor and the nutrients are in the water, which has become soup stock. The transfer of nutrients from meat to water also occurs in stews. As long as the liquid used in boiling is a part of the dish the nutrients are not lost. But don't boil food and then throw the valuable water away.

Steaming

This is the best alternative to boiling when you want to cook vegetables (or even meat) without using the water as part of a sauce. You can buy a steamer, or make your own by placing the vegetable in a strainer or wire basket that does not touch the top of the water in the pot. Cover, boil the water, and you will have tender vegetables that retain most of their vitamins and minerals.

Even with steaming, some of the vitamins do get into the water. Therefore, I suggest that you save this water (in a tightly covered jar in the refrigerator) and use it later for making a sauce or soup. You can concentrate it by using it over and over each time you steam a vegetable, but it should be used for a sauce or soup within a week, or it will spoil.

Braising

This term is used to describe a process in which you simmer food in a very small amount of liquid that will later become the sauce or gravy for the dish. It is an excellent way of preparing food, as long as you use the Fat-Free Trick to get rid of any fat that floats to the top. The liquid can then be thickened with flour, cornstarch, arrowroot or a *buerre manie* (mixture of flour and polyunsaturated margarine), or with a low-fat milk powder if you want to make a "cream" sauce.

The few cooking methods described in this section can make your meals more nutritious, more flavorful, and far less fatty.

I hope these tips are helpful. For even more ideas on low-fat cooking—including plenty of recipes—consult any of the cookbooks in the following list. Since I first introduced the low-fat, low-cholesterol diet in the 1940s, many creative cooks have adapted it to all types of cuisine, from gourmet to Mexican to Jewish. By using this chapter and one or more of these books,

I'm sure you'll find that low-fat eating doesn't have to be low in flavor or interest.

Low-Fat, Low-Cholesterol Cookbooks

Aulicino, Armand. *The New International Cuisine.* New York: A & W Publishers, 1979.

Bennett, Iva, and Simon, Martha. *The Prudent Diet.* New York: David White, 1973.

Betz, Eleanor P. *Holiday Eating for a Healthy Heart.* Chicago: Rush, Presby, St. Luke's, 1981.

————. *Summertime Eating for a Healthy Heart: Cook Out—Eat Out the Low Cholesterol Way.* Chicago: Rush, Presby, St. Luke's, 1981.

Bond, Clara-Beth Young, et al. *Low Fat, Low Cholesterol Diet.* Garden City, N.Y.: Doubleday, 1971.

Brown, W. J., et al. *Cook to Your Heart's Content: On a Low-Fat, Low-Salt Diet.* New York: Van Nostrand Reinhold, 1976.

Carper, Jean, and Eyton, Audrey. *The Revolutionary Seven-Unit Low-Fat Diet.* New York: Rawson Wade, 1981.

Caviani, Mable. *Low Cholesterol Cooking: A Collection of Regional and Ethnic Recipes.* Chicago: Contemporary Books, 1981.

Cholesterol Diet Cookbook. Miami: Merit Publications, 1974.

Claiborne, Craig. *Craig Claiborne's Gourmet Diet.* New York: Times Books, 1980.

Cutler, Carol. *Haute Cuisine for Your Heart's Delight; a Low-Cholesterol Cookbook for Gourmets.* New York: C. N. Potter, 1973.

Dosti, Rose. *Light Style: The New American Cuisine. The Low Calorie, Low Salt, Low Fat Way to Good Food and Good Health.* New York: Harper & Row, 1979.

Eshleman, Ruthe, and Winston, Mary. *The American Heart Association Cookbook.* New York: David McKay, 1979.

Evans, D. Wainwright, and Greenfield, Meta A. *Cooking for Your Heart's Content.* New York: Paddington Press, 1977.

Faigel, Frayda. *The Happy Heart Cookbook.* Westport, Ct.: Condor Publishing Co., 1977.

Forsythe, Elizabeth. *The Low-Fat Gourmet.* London: Michael Joseph, 1981.

Gibbons, Barbara. *Lean Cuisine.* New York: Harper & Row, 1979.

Grace, Vilma J. *Latin American and Cholesterol Conscious Cooking.* Washington, D.C.: Acropolis, 1979.

Guerard, Michel. *Michel Guerard's Cuisine Minceur.* New York: William Morrow, 1976.

Havenstein, Nathalie, and Richardson, Elizabeth. *The Anti-Coronary Cookbook; How to Achieve Weight Reduction and Cholesterol Control.* Sydney: Ure Smith, 1969.

Jencks, Tina. *In Good Taste.* Berkeley, Calif.: Lancaster-Miller Publishers, 1980.

Jones, Jeanne. *Diet for a Happy Heart.* San Francisco: 101 Productions, 1975.

Jones, Suzanne. *The Low-Cholesterol Food Processor Cookbook.* New York: Doubleday, 1980.

Lampen, Nevada. *Fat-Free Recipes.* Salem, N.H.: Faber and Faber, 1977.

Leinwoll, Stanley. *Low Cholesterol, Lower Calorie Desserts.* New York: Scribner's, 1973.

———. *Low Cholesterol, Lower Calorie French Cooking.* New York: Scribner's, 1974.

McFarlane, Helen B. *The Cholesterol Control Cookbook.* New York: Baronet, 1977.

Mac Rae, Norma M. *How to Have Your Cake and Eat It Too! Diet Cooking for the Whole Family: Diabetic, Hypoglycemic, Low Cholesterol, Low Fat, Low Salt, Low Calorie Diets.* Edmonds, Wash.: Alaska Northwest, 1975.

Margie, Joyce Daly, et al. *Living Better: Recipes for a Healthy Heart.* Radnor, Pa.: Chilton, 1980.

Payne, Alma, and Callahan, Dorothy. *The Fat and Sodium Control Cookbook: A Handy and Authoritative Guide for Those on Sodium-Restricted or Fat-Controlled Diets—Including Suggestions for Controlling Carbohydrate, Cholesterol and Saturated Fats.* Boston: Little, Brown, 1975.

Rosenthal, Sylvia Divorsky. *Live High on Low Fat.* New York: J. B. Lippincott, 1975.

Roth, June. *Low-Cholesterol Jewish Cookery: The Unsaturated Fat Way.* New York: Arco, 1978.

Skinner, Mildred. *Low Cholesterol Cookbook: Doctor Approved.* San Antonio: Naylor, 1975.

Stead, Evelyn, and Warren, Gloria. *Low-Fat Cookery.* New York: McGraw-Hill, 1977.

Stern, Ellen, and Michaels, Jonathan. *The Good Heart Diet Cookbook.* New Haven, Conn.: Ticknor and Fields, 1982.

Wade, Carlson. *The Low Fat Meat and Poultry Cookbook.* New York: Drake Publishing Co., 1973.

Wayne, Doreen. *The Healthy Gourmet: Low Calorie—Low Cholesterol—Low Cost Cookery.* Woodstock, N.Y.: Beekman Publishers, 1979.

Weiss, Elizabeth S., and Wolfson, Rita Parsont. *Cholesterol Counter.* New York: Pyramid Books, 1973.

―――. *The Gourmet's Low Cholesterol Cookbook.* New York: Pyramid Books, 1973.

Whyte, H. M. *Eat to Your Heart's Content.* New York: Hawthorn Books, 1962.

Zane, Polly. *The Jack Sprat Cookbook or Good Eating on a Low Cholesterol Diet.* New York: Harper & Row, 1973.

Zugibe, Frederick Thomas. *Eat, Drink, and Lower Your Cholesterol.* New York: McGraw-Hill, 1963.

Chapter 7

EXERCISE— YOUR RIGHT

Exercise is good for you. What else is new?

Anyone who hasn't been trapped at the bottom of a mine shaft for the last ten years knows that there's an exercise craze going on. Streets that used to be seen only by milkmen at 6 A.M. now are crowded with joggers. The leotard and running-shoe businesses are booming. Jack LaLanne and Richard Simmons are making fortunes and becoming folk heroes. The word "fit," which frequently used to be associated with clothes that were the right size for the body, now commonly refers to good health. However, there's one problem with exercise in the view of many people—it's boring.

That's the chief complaint people make about exercise, and of course it's the same gripe they have about dieting. Who wants to lie on the floor and wave his arms and legs in the air for fifteen minutes each day? Who wants to eat celery and broiled fish all the time?

But like a diet, an exercise program doesn't have to be a duty or something you force yourself to do. It doesn't even have to be a plodding step you take on the long road to a barely discernible goal. Exercise is a *right*. You have a right to be as healthy as possible, and you have a right to the enjoyable pur-

151

suit of that health (which is very much like the pursuit of happiness). You also have a right to eat 2 pounds of butter a day and spend most of your waking hours sitting in front of a television set drinking beer. But by now it should be obvious that the rights to good diet and adequate exercise are the right rights to exercise.

This play on words is merely an attention-getting way of pointing out that the attainment of health is your choice. If you've chosen (as I assume you have, since you're reading this book) to exercise your right to the best health you can obtain, then you should know that it's also your right to make the obtaining of that health as interesting and enjoyable as you can. Getting there can be *at least* half of the fun.

I hope I've already convinced you that diets can be varied, interesting and enjoyable as well as noticeably rewarding. Now I'm going to show you that the same can be true of exercise.

What's in It for You?

It never hurts to take a look at the rewards first. You've probably heard all about the benefits of physical activity, but there may be some you've missed—and examining the prizes is good for motivation.

Exercise can make you more energetic. Surprised? Maybe you thought that exercise just naturally wears you out, especially if you're not used to it. Wrong. The main thing that tires people out is *stress,* and exercise relieves stress.

Stress creates tension—it tightens your muscles and constricts your blood vessels, making it harder for blood (which carries oxygen to every part of your body) to get through. Exercise puts your muscles to work performing physical tasks, so they loosen up instead of being tense and tight. It makes your heart pump harder, which forces oxygen-carrying blood through your veins and arteries. It makes you breathe faster, so you take in more oxygen. And that extra oxygen goes to your brain and other tissues and peps you up.

You know that the calories you take in will either be used as energy or stored as fat. The fat that makes you look unattractive and endangers your arteries is just energy waiting to be used. Exercise acts as a catalyst or activator, waking up that sleeping energy and putting it to work. You have the energy—it's been there all along; it just needs a little booster to get started in the right direction.

You may feel exhausted when you've finished an exercise session, especially if you're not used to it. But after a little rest to allow your startled body functions to regroup, you'll find that you're ready for more. And the stress that has been making you tense will have been worked off.

Chronic stress has not only been implicated as a causative factor in high blood pressure, it has been tried and convicted. People who work under stressful conditions, or who allow personal problems to make them worry most of the time, have a greater incidence of high blood pressure than do people who direct their natural energies elsewhere—and high blood pressure leads to more serious heart disease. Of course, we can't all control the conditions under which we work and live or wave off our personal problems. But we can use exercise to reduce the amount of stress those conditions or problems cause.

Exercise can make you look better. This is one of the obvious benefits of exercise. Exercise takes the energy that has been masquerading as fat and turns it to a useful purpose. You lose the fat, your muscles become toned and firm, your posture improves and you can wear designer jeans that fit because you are fit.

Exercise even improves the look in your eyes—because you have more energy, your eyes become brighter, more alert and even "sparkly." Your skin looks better because it's not flabby, and the extra oxygen you get adds color to your cheeks. It's a lot easier to smile when your facial muscles are limber than when they're tight and tense.

When you look better naturally, you automatically start paying more attention to your appearance, and pretty soon you look better all over. You don't need me to tell you that—your mirror and your friends will let you know.

Exercise reduces your risk of heart disease. A twenty-year test conducted by Stanford University epidemiologist Ralph Paffenbarger, M.D., Ph.D., makes this point. He studied about 17,000 men between the ages of 35 and 74, the ages when heart attacks are most likely to occur. Over ten years, he found that men who had made sure to get regular exercise throughout their lives had at least 50 percent *fewer* heart attacks than men who spent most of their time in chairs—and this applied even to men who were cigarette smokers, men who were overweight, men who had high blood pressure and men who had the uncontrollable risk factor of heart disease in their families.

Dr. Paffenbarger's work is only one example of a fact nobody disputes any more: Active people are less likely to have heart attacks than inactive people. Exercise is a weapon.

Exercise increases your stamina. That simply means that exercise makes you stronger, which is obvious when you look at the muscular bodies of weight lifters or the legs of ballerinas. Remember the old ads about the 98-pound weakling who got sand kicked in his face until he took the Charles Atlas body-building course?

These examples are extremes, but the basic principle applies to everyone. After a while, your body gets used to exercise. It "learns" to perform more and more physical activity, just as your mind learns to solve more and more difficult mathematical problems as you go from grade to grade in school. But you don't have to become a Ph.D. in exercise; your individual lifestyle will tell you whether you're ready to graduate to more strenuous exercise or stay at the same level of exertion, feeling better and stronger in either case than you ever did before your muscles became educated.

Exercise makes you feel better about yourself. It's no secret that people who look good, have high energy levels and feel strong have much better mental outlooks than those who look fat or flabby, are tired all the time and feel weak. We know exercise is good, and when we know we're doing something good, the knowledge fills us with a natural pride—not false pride or the kind that goes before a fall, but *real* pride, the kind that goes before the warm glow of self-confidence.

Exercise helps to lengthen your life. One of the first realizations of the connection between exercise and long life grew out of a heart-attack study among bus employees in England. Researchers discovered that bus drivers (who sat down all day) had a far greater incidence of heart attacks—40 percent of which were fatal—than did bus conductors (who were on their feet all day collecting fares from passengers). The conductors not only walked back and forth in the buses, they had to climb stairs, since the study was done in London, where the buses are double-decker!

Later, similar studies compared sedentary office workers with stevedores, railroad workers and other manual laborers. They all confirmed the fact that vigorous physical exercise, as a lifetime habit, contributes to a long life.

Office workers don't have to despair, however, and the popularity of health clubs proves that a lot of them don't. Even in New York City, where there are more sit-down workers and fewer open spaces than anywhere else, the exercise craze is booming. Indoor swimming pools, racquetball courts and gymnasia are packed to overflowing at lunch hour and in the early evening. Central Park has more joggers than muggers in the early morning. Jogging tracks are even replacing singles bars as places for couples to meet—and the couples aren't all young.

No matter where you live or what kind of work you do, you can increase your chances for a longer life by keeping your body in motion.

Exercise increases your HDL level and lowers your LDL level. You may have thought I was getting off the subject of arteriosclerosis, but that's not so. The health of your arteries is, after all, the main subject of this book and the focus of my life's work. In the course of that work I have been impressed and delighted by the statistics that show blood levels of protective HDL going up after exercise, while dangerous LDL levels go down.

Triglyceride levels have also been shown to improve, and it is thought that exercise slows down the clotting time of blood. These factors make it less likely that an active person will suffer from the degenerative diseases that lead to arteriosclerosis, heart attack and stroke, and more likely that the same active person will live longer than his sedentary friend.

Those are the rewards of exercise—certainly worth striving for, in anyone's book. But what about the drawbacks?

Making Exercise Fun

The complaint that exercise is boring is hard to argue against if you're talking to someone who thinks of it only in terms of calisthenics and rooms full of people all doing the same movements over and over again. But that's only one side of the exercise coin. The other side has three faces, described by three words you may never have connected with the word "exercise." They are "dancing," "transportation," and "sport."

Dancing. If you think dancing is only for teenagers at the prom, you're out of step.

Whatever your age, there was a dance popular in your youth that's still popular today, because today anything goes. Whether you Charleston, rumba, jitterbug, twist, cha-cha, frug, disco or boogaloo, your dance is *in*—and it's good exercise. Rock bands, jazz bands, mellow bands and big bands can be heard everywhere, and if you can hear it, you can dance to it.

You can dance almost anywhere, including the privacy of your own home. You can take the floor with a partner, a crowd or alone. You can go out and dance to a live band, dance to recorded music at a disco, or dance to your radio or tape deck at home.

If more structured dancing is to your liking, you can take classes in square dancing, aerobics, acrobatics, jazz, modern dance, or classical ballet—even hula dancing or belly dancing if you like something a bit out of the ordinary. You don't have to be young, and you don't even have to be good at it; the rewards are the fun you have and the exercise you give to your body.

Transportation. All of us have to get from one place to another, but does it have to be in a car?

Americans are car-happy, as evidenced by the fact that our streets and highways remain overcrowded in spite of the inflated price of gas. But did you know that walking is one of the best exercises you can perform?

Interestingly, the place where people walk the most is the previously mentioned place where workers sit the most— New York City. The truck and taxi traffic is so heavy, and parking places so expensive and hard to find, that most New Yorkers don't even own cars. For long distances they ride the taxis and subways, but for medium and short distances, they walk.

Californians, at the opposite extreme, practically live in their cars. Where the New Yorker will walk fifteen blocks to buy a newspaper and exercise his dog, the Californian will drive two blocks and let his dog out in the back yard.

Why then, you may ask, is the typical Californian a picture of health who looks like a bronzed god or goddess in a suntan-oil ad? Because the warm climate in that state encourages people to seek forms of exercise other than walking. When Californians drive, it's often to sun-drenched tennis courts, golf courses and beaches—and an awful lot of them have swimming pools right in their back yards that are used for daily exercise. Californians are also known for their love of "health foods," most of which are extremely low in saturated fat, so the people from the Golden State stay pretty healthy even without walking. Just living there doesn't do the work for them—you can get a gorgeous tan by lying on your back all day, but you will not receive the benefit of the exercise that contributes to good looks and good health.

Where do you fit in this picture? It doesn't really matter where you live. Do you automatically jump into the car when you need an item from a store or want to visit a friend? Or do you stop to think about how far away that store or friend is located and consider the possibility of making the trip on foot?

Come to think of it, how far is your home from your place of work?—from the dry cleaner?—the newsstand?—the movie theater?—your church or temple?—the library?

If all those places are too far away for walking, what about bicycling or—for those of us who are really adventurous and want to keep up with the times—roller skating? Both will get you where you want to go, save you the price of gas, help to keep the air free of pollution and, most important, give your body a good physical workout without making you think you're exercising.

The point is to stay out of the car—and that includes mopeds, motorcycles, golf carts, snowmobiles and dune buggies. Get on your feet or pedal a bicycle; it's good for you as well as for the environment.

Sport. This is the category that takes the "boring" out of exercise for many people—especially if you are not fond of dancing, are in too much of a hurry to walk and need the added mental stimulus of competition. There's an ideal sport for almost everyone.

Are you a loner? Swimming may be for you; it's a sport that exercises every muscle in your body. Are you a born team member? Join a volleyball or softball team. Is playing one-on-one more to your liking? Go out for tennis or racquetball. Do you want a more leisurely form of exercise? Try golf—without the cart.

No matter what your preferences—whether you want to be indoors or out, alone or with other people—there is some form of sport that can bring you all the rewards mentioned earlier in this chapter, along with a good measure of fun.

"But I Don't Have Time"

That's the second most common complaint about exercise. But when you consider the benefits of activity against the penalties of being lethargic, the truth is that you don't have time *not* to exercise. Being inactive may add minutes to your day, but it can subtract years from your life.

Being busy is a way to take the "boring" out of even the most monotonous exercises. Does the thought of standard exercises make you groan? Then do something else at the same time, something you would otherwise do while sitting or standing still.

You can talk on the phone while doing leg-lifts. You can read while riding a stationary bicycle. You can figure out a problem or compose a letter while jogging or doing sit-ups. You can jump rope while watching the evening news (or a soap opera) on television.

All the excuses are just excuses, after all. You can gossip or discuss a business strategy while working out with a friend or colleague. You *can* do it—if you want to.

Is There Anyone Who Shouldn't Exercise?

Probably not. Exercise includes such a wide range of activity that there is literally something for almost everyone, and I say "almost" only because there's always the possibility of an exception to the rule. But if there is someone who really shouldn't exercise at all, I don't know who he or she might be.

The type of exercise is a different matter. Exercise, like diet, has to be tailored to the individual. As a general rule, the younger and healthier you are when you start your exercise program, the more strenuous your activity can be. But that's only a general rule.

Learn your needs and your tolerance. The question of exercise should be brought up when you see your doctor to learn what your blood-lipid levels are. Ask how much exercise you need for weight loss (if any) and how much for maintenance of a healthy cardiovascular system—that is, to keep your pulse and breathing at their uppermost level of efficiency and your blood pressure down.

The doctor will take a number of factors into consideration: your age, weight, current level of activity and any pre-existing health problems you may have. He may suggest or administer an endurance test to see how your system reacts to unexpected bursts of activity.

Do not, under any circumstances, begin a sudden program of strenuous activity without checking with your doctor first. There are hidden diseases (for example, diabetes) that can be aggravated by sudden changes in activity levels. It could be that your blood pressure is already too high (another silent disease) or that you have cardiovascular problems that have not yet made themselves known through symptoms. By checking your history and making some tests, your doctor will be able to determine how much exercise will be good for you, and how much could be harmful.

You have to begin an exercise program slowly, especially if you are in your middle or late years (that is, over 35) and are not used to a lot of activity. A sudden jolt is not good, and can be bad. Even professional athletes know that they have to warm up gradually before engaging in strenuous activity—and who is more accustomed to it than they?

Recipes for Exercise

Here are some suggestions for exercises—you could think of them as exercise "recipes"—that you may find helpful once your doctor has determined how much activity you should take on, and how fast. At the Institute, we call these "preventive" exercises, since we know they contribute to the prevention of heart disease, premature aging and early death. They have a double purpose:

1. To raise your heart rate to its optimum level for physiologic safety, comfort and benefit
2. To prevent degenerative diseases and premature aging

Warming-Up Exercise

Toe-Touching. Stand up straight with your feet 12 to 24 inches apart. Bend over and attempt to touch your toes with your fingertips.

You probably won't be able to do it at first—at least not with your knees straight. But that's not the point. The point is to try. As you bend and reach, your muscles start getting the idea that they're being asked to do something unfamiliar. Don't try to force them; if you do, they'll rebel by causing you pain.

Reach down as far as you can comfortably, then bend your knees (to relieve pressure on your lower back as you stand up), straighten up and place your hands on your hips. Then try again. That's all there is to it.

That's all there is to the effort, but the results are something else again. Each time you reach for your toes, you will gradually get a little bit closer; you may not notice a decrease in the distance with each bend, but by the fifth try, your fingers should be going lower than they did at first.

Other things will be happening, too. Your muscles will be loosening (gradually, not dramatically), and your heart and lungs will be working just a little bit harder than they did before you started. If you toe-touch so quickly that you end up gasping for breath, you're going too fast. Take it easy, and be gentle with yourself.

Start out with five toe-touching attempts. The next day go for six, then seven, and keep increasing by one try each day. By the time you get up to fifty, you probably will have those toes well in hand, and many people even reach the point at which they can place their hands flat on the floor without bending their knees. But that's Olympic gold medal territory—reach as far as you can reach *comfortably,* and don't try to be a superstar.

This warm-up exercise benefits your heart, lungs, brain, spine, arm and leg muscles and abdomen. Once you've completed your daily number of toe-touches, your body will be ready to move on to something a little more strenuous.

The Workout

The Upside-down Bicycle. Now that you are warmed up, lie flat on your back on the floor, raise your legs in the air and begin to pedal an imaginary upside-down bicycle. Pump your pedaling legs as vigorously as you would if you were riding a real bike.

Next, and while still pedaling, massage your abdomen with one hand, moving the hand in a clockwise direction and keeping in rhythm with your pedaling. (I'll tell you in a few pages why the massage is good for you.)

For the first few days, try to keep this exercise going for three or four minutes, but stop if you feel yourself getting tired. Increase your time gradually each day until you've reached about 100 pedals—you will have "biked" along the road to better health.

After you've gotten used to the pedaling and massaging, add head-turning to this exercise: As you pedal and massage your abdomen, turn your head from side to side, breathing deeply, slowly and rhythmically. When you stop, slow down gradually; otherwise you may feel dizzy when you get up because so much blood is still being pumped to your legs. You will be exercising your legs, thighs, hips, abdomen, neck, lungs and heart all at the same time!

The Semi-Headstand. Lie on the floor and rest after bicycling, until your breathing has returned to normal and you feel relaxed. Then raise your legs again, this time also raising your hips in the air. Place your hands under your hips to brace them, with your elbows and upper arms flat on the floor. Your weight will be supported by your shoulders and elbows.

Bend your knees, and bring them as close to your forehead as you can—you are almost standing on your head! Then straighten your legs out, and spread them wide out to your sides. Bring them back together (as if they were the blades of a pair of scissors), then bend the knees again and bring them back to your head.

Try to do this exercise five times at first, then increase by one or more times each day until you feel you have reached your limit.

At first it probably won't be easy to do it even once, and you'll certainly feel the pull in your thigh muscles as you spread your legs to open the "scissors." But don't feel bad—nobody's keeping score. After a few tries it will become easier and easier, and soon you'll be able to add head-turns just as you did with the upside-down bicycle. Turn your head from side to side with each leg movement, and breathe deeply.

This excellent exercise, once mastered, limbers the same muscles as the bicycle maneuver does (only more so) and also acts to actively pump the blood from your lower body up through your neck and into your brain.

The Frog. If you've ever watched a frog hop from one lily pad to another, you may feel like one while doing this exercise. If you feel ridiculous, laugh at yourself; that's good exercise, too.

Stand straight and start to jump straight up—just a little jump at first, then gradually higher until you're as high as you want to get.

Then jump to the left. Jump back to your starting spot. Jump to the right. Jump back to the starting spot. Each spot is a lily pad, and you are a frog.

Once you have that pattern down pat, swing your arms out in front of you with the first jump. As you jump to the side, swing your arms out to the sides. When you return to your starting "pad," bring your arms out in front again. You've never seen a frog pull off a maneuver like that!

Is there something you need on the other side of the room? Don't walk over to get it, jump! Is the phone ringing? Hop to it! This exercise increases your heartbeat and makes you breathe faster and more deeply, which are the basic points of the "aerobic" method of exercise devised by Kenneth Cooper, M.D., of the Cooper Clinic in Dallas. Aerobics are superior exercises that gradually increase the working capacity of your heart and lungs and keep energy-rich oxygen circulating throughout your body; other aerobic exercises include jogging, swimming, jumping rope and cross-country skiing.

How long should you jump around like a restless frog? Only about five or six jumps on the first day, then a few more each day until you are used to the exercise and are comfortable doing it. Don't try to overdo it—that can damage both your body and your motivation. By increasing the number of your jumps gradually, you can eventually reach a point at which you can jump (with or without a rope) for ten or fifteen minutes a day. When this level is reached you should be able to get your heart rate up to about 120 beats per minute, which is considered ideal in the aerobic plan. Later in this chapter I'll tell you how to take your pulse, and explain how important it is to "wind down" gradually after having increased your pulse to 120.

Yes and No. These simple exercises can be done individually or along with almost any of the others, once you've become accomplished enough to have mastered the basics and want some variation. They improve the circulation of blood through the carotid arteries in your neck, which lead directly to your brain.

Breathing deeply, first rotate your head in a clockwise direction. Stop, then rotate in a counterclockwise direction. Try fifteen to twenty rotations each way.

Next do the "yes" exercise, moving your head and neck forward and backward as far as they will go, as if you were nodding an affirmative answer to a question. Do this one fifteen or twenty times, and remember to keep breathing deeply all the while.

After "yes" comes "no." Turn your head and neck from side to side as vigorously as you can, as if trying to convince a deaf person that you mean business when you say "no."

It's important to remember to move your eyes in the same direction as your head; if you try to focus on one spot as your head moves, you'll get dizzy. So look around, up and down, and from side to side as you exercise (you may discover that the ceiling needs painting).

With these exercises you are increasing the flow of blood to your brain, as well as keeping that blood active—just as a rolling stone gathers no moss, rapidly circulating blood gathers (almost) no clots. I had to add "almost" because there are other factors involved that can produce clots even when circulation is good; but these exercises are excellent preventive measures, and your diet along with the Institute Formula should take care of most of the other clotting and plaquing factors.

Sit-ups. Everybody knows what sit-ups are all about; they are especially good for anyone who has a protruding abdomen (more commonly called a "tummy" or a "potbelly").

Lie flat on your back on the floor, with your arms extended over your head. Then sit up (slowly at first), and reach for your toes. (You may want to start out with a simpler version, only raising your shoulders off the floor.)

At first you'll probably find it easier to do this with your knees bent. But as you get used to it, as your muscles limber up and your strength increases, you'll find that you can do it with your legs straight—and eventually, you should be able to grab your toes.

Start with just four or five sit-ups, then increase them by one or two each day. After a while you'll be doing them regularly, and your pulse will be getting up to the desired 120 beats per minute.

Internal Massage. Most exercise programs concentrate on the development of the back and abdominal muscles. I want you to take care of your vital internal organs as well. These—especially your aorta (the main artery)—age far more rapidly than any muscle.

Lie on your back, raise your bent knees, and massage your abdomen with one hand, just as you did in the upside-down bicycle exercise. Begin gently, moving your hand in a clockwise direction, then gradually exert more pressure. You are coming as close as you can get to reaching inside your body and massaging your internal organs.

This massage will stimulate the circulation to those organs, helping them to function more efficiently. Breathe deeply all during the massage.

Push-ups. We all know the Army uses push-ups as punishment, but you should think instead of the rewards they're providing for your entire body. The soldiers get the same rewards, of course, but probably don't think of anything except how much they hate the sergeant.

Lie flat on the floor, face down, with the palms of your hands flat out at shoulder level. Then raise your body up on your outstretched arms while breathing deeply and consciously hardening your abdominal muscles.

Like many people, you probably won't be able to do a push-up at all at first. Push-ups are hard to do, which just makes it all the more satisfying the first time you accomplish a complete one.

Don't try *too* hard. Attempt one or two push-ups the first day, then keep trying until you have achieved two complete ones. Next add a third. After that, it will get easier and easier, trust me. But increase the number gradually, never pushing yourself to the point of straining. Even when you've conquered the task, don't let your pulse rate exceed 120, and stop if you start to feel fatigued or sore. Depending upon your sex, age and condition at the beginning of your exercise program, five to twenty-five push-ups a day (without strain) is a good goal for adults. Remember, those soldiers are kids just out of high school!

Lift the World. Archimedes said that he could lift the world if only he had the proper base. Your body is your world, and you *do* have the proper base—you're standing on it. You can lift your personal world with the familiar old exercise called knee bends.

Start with a partial squat, keeping your buttocks above the level of your knees, and raise your arms straight out in front of you. Then stand up. Go a step farther—raise yourself up on your toes. Then lower yourself to the flat-footed position, and squat again. That's all there is to it.

The catch is that it may be hard to keep your balance at first. But don't worry about it; it happens to almost every beginner. If you fall off to the side, just pick yourself up, take a deep breath, and start over, maybe with a little help.

Ballet students do this exercise all the time, using a bar on the wall for balance. You don't have to have a bar installed in your home—use a chair or the edge of a table. Helping yourself in this way is not considered cheating.

Start out with two or three world-lifts a day, then increase gradually as you get stronger. Ten to fifty a day makes a good goal, depending on your endurance. This is the toughest, yet the best exercise for your heart and circulation, not to mention the rest of you.

Going up on your toes has a purpose of its own, by the way. This movement stimulates the circulation in your feet, ankles and legs, which helps to prevent such conditions as varicose veins, arteriosclerosis of the leg arteries and even arthritis. You can apply this motion to several of the other exercises once you've gotten the hang of the basic movements.

Standing on tip-toe is particularly helpful to people whose lives are basically sedentary—that is, those who sit at a desk all day, drive for a living or stand in the same spot without moving around a lot. Your legs were designed for moving you around—if you can't move forward, move up!

Winding-down Exercises

Winding down is just as important as warming up. If you start vigorous exercise suddenly, it's a severe shock to the body that is used to a sedentary state. Likewise, once the body gets into the rhythm and pattern of exercise, it's a similar jolt to just quit cold turkey without any warning. Both starting and stopping have to be gradual.

When you've finished the last exercise you plan to do, just stand there and walk in place for about two minutes, gradually going from a brisk pace to a slow pace. When you're going so slowly that the next step is stopping, stop. Your pulse and breathing will have been slowing down gradually as you decrease your speed, and, while they will still be faster than normal for a few minutes, they will be moving downward.

Taking Your Pulse

Take your pulse by placing the first three fingers of one hand on the radial artery of the opposite wrist; the palm should be facing up. (To find the radial artery—where the pulse is strongest—think of an imaginary line extending from your index finger down to your wrist.)

Take the pulse while looking at a stopwatch or clock that has a sweep second hand (or a digital clock that shows the seconds). Start counting at the beginning of a minute and continue until a full minute has passed. The number you've reached at the end of one minute is your pulse rate *at that moment.*

Your normal pulse will change many times during a day, so don't be upset if it's not always the same—it should vary within a normal *range.*

The normal range for most adults is 60 to 80 beats per minute at rest. During exercise it's good to increase the number of beats to around 120, after which it should go back to about

60 to 80. There are exceptions, however—some marathon runners and Olympic athletes have normal pulse rates as low as 40 beats per minute at rest; other normal individuals have been found to have rates as fast as 100 without any illness at all. But these are unusual; chances are your resting pulse will fall somewhere in the 60-to-80 range.

All these "recipes" have been for the types of exercises that a lot of people consider "boring." If you just can't stand them, forget them. Join a dance club or class, or take a closer look at the transportation and sport categories of exercise.

Your Feet Were Made for Walking

What does walking do for you? What can it do for you if you're not already an habitual walker? Let's take a look at what it's done for some famous walkers of the past; it won't make you a Nobel Prize winner or a President, but it can make you a far healthier and happier person in any level of life.

The value of walking for health was first described by Hippocrates, the father of medicine, in the fourth century B.C. He urged walking for daily exercise as well as for sport. Later, in the thirteenth century, Dante Alighieri spoke passionately of his long walks in search of his Beatrice as he composed his immortal poetry the *Divine Comedy.*

Charles Darwin in the mid-nineteenth century walked the countryside for his ailing health as he pondered the *Origin of Species.* Ludwig van Beethoven, who was known for taking long walks in the country, was musically inspired by his communication with nature. In 1880, Bismarck of Germany took his dogs along for long walks in the forests as he evolved decisions that would affect the fates of Germany, France and all Europe.

Other renowned persons such as Benjamin Franklin, Thomas Jefferson and Robert Louis Stevenson were noted for their long "health walks," while Nobel Laureate Thomas Mann, who took long walks paced by his intelligent dog, wrote a famous essay on walking for countless other followers of good health.

In more recent times, President Harry S. Truman became famous for his daily "constitutionals," which must have had at least an inadvertent effect on the constitutions of the Secret Service agents who had to follow him everywhere he went. If you take up walking for exercise, sport or pure pleasure, you will find yourself in very prestigious company.

Here's how to walk to your best advantage: Keep your lower back straight, walking as "tall" as possible. Hold your shoulders back, your chest out and your chin up, breathing deeply, rhythmically and slowly.

Many people pace themselves by walking to music, whether it's an imaginary tune heard only in their heads, or actual music heard through earphones attached to a lightweight portable radio or tape deck. If you have the tape apparatus, you can set your own pace by playing a tape of a Sousa march, a Bach fugue or a Fleetwood Mac song—whatever suits your fancy.

Walk as often as possible, climb stairs whenever you have the chance, move around instead of sitting still. When walking, wear comfortable shoes and casual, loose-fitting clothes, and walk in the most pleasant environment you can find. Walking can be fun!

Swimming—the All-Around Sport

Swimming is at the top of the list for exercise benefits. Your heat, lungs and virtually all the muscles in your body are brought into play. In addition, swimming is refreshing, relaxing, healthfully tiring and exhilarating.

My favorite swimmer is my friend Martha Feuchtwanger (widow of the noted writer Leon Feuchtwanger) who, at this writing, is 91 years old, and an ideal example of fitness. She has been an ocean swimmer for seventy years, and up until two years ago swam daily throughout the year in the Pacific Ocean. This exercise is certainly largely responsible for the fact that, at her advanced age, she is fit, productive and most active in Los Angeles cultural life.

A poor climate is no excuse for not swimming, since there are indoor pools and swimming clubs everywhere. And the old wives' tale that women shouldn't swim during their menstrual periods is nonsense; there would be no women's Olympic swimming contests if that were true. The only valid excuse for not swimming is that you don't like it—in which case, there are plenty of other types of exercise from which you can choose.

The Running Madness

Running has become so popular that the Boston Marathon, which used to attract a hundred or so contestants, last year started off with thousands of people in shorts and tank tops jostling each other for the privilege of running over twenty-six miles without stopping! I wouldn't prescribe a workout like that for most people—it takes an extraordinary constitution and a great deal of long, arduous training to get yourself in the proper condition for such a run. The marathon runners are amateurs, but they have to train as hard and as often as professional athletes to get in shape.

For most of us, daily jogging on a much more casual level is beneficial, stimulating and, for many, fun—especially in the company of others. Joggers talk about the "high" they get from running, which is the effect of superior oxygen consumption, and increased heartbeat and the release of certain chemicals which contribute to well-being.

Jogging is excellent exercise for the right people, but you must not just take off and start running around the block without the guidance of a physician—especially if you are more than 35 years old. That's not to say that it's dangerous; it just has to be regulated. Many people jog after having had heart attacks, and it's not unusual to see a person of 70, 80 or 90 years of age jogging along. But at the risk of sounding like a broken record, I urge you to see your doctor *before* you start jogging so you won't have to see him as a result of it.

To make exercise work for you, practice it regularly, but don't become a fitness fanatic. Exercise should be a pleasure, not a grim task. Work gently toward the goal of getting your pulse up to 120 beats per minute during a workout. Be sure to warm up gradually and wind down gradually after each exercise session. Develop the habit of breathing deeply and rhythmically as you exercise. Stretch as often during the day as you can.

Assuredly, regular exercise can help you live healthfully and live longer. Try it (if you haven't already). You may be amazed and delighted at what this segment of the Institute Program—combined with the Institute Formula and an individualized low-saturated-fat diet—can do for you!

Chapter 8

ALCOHOL, CAFFEINE AND TOBACCO— A TRIPLE THREAT YOU CAN HANDLE

Anyone who picks up a health book is likely to think, "Right off the bat this doctor is going to tell me to quit drinking and smoking." No, not this doctor.

Drinking (which most people take to mean drinking alcoholic beverages) and smoking are such deeply established habits in the lives of many people that quitting would be absolute misery. And it's certainly not my goal to make your life miserable or to make anyone feel that good health is not worth the price you have to pay. If drinking and smoking are pleasures in your life, then it's possible to keep these habits and still be healthy, which is sort of like having your cake and eating it, too.

How is this possible? It's simply a matter of putting that key word "moderation" to practical use. Overdoing anything is harmful; overdoing your use of alcohol and cigarettes can be *very* harmful, or even fatal. Therefore, it's not alcohol and tobacco that are forbidden in the Institute Program, it's overdoing.

Alcohol

Is alcohol a blessing? Often.

Is alcohol a curse? Same answer.

Is alcohol here to stay? Definitely.

The failure of Prohibition back in the 20s showed us how futile it was to try to outlaw alcohol. People who wanted to drink did so anyway, illegal or not. Even if you're too young to remember that time, you've heard stories about speakeasies, bathtub gin and the takeover of the alcoholic beverage industry by organized crime. The liquor was still there, but instead of buying it from licensed stores, people bought it from gangsters—and the gangsters made a fortune!

Today, Americans spend about 43 billion dollars a year on alcoholic beverages—both paying for the liquor itself and then paying for all the problems it causes—and that figure is rising all the time. The truth is that we spend more on alcohol than we do on our health. More than 65 percent of the U.S. population drinks alcohol: Of men who drink, 39 percent are occasional drinkers, and 61 percent are moderate or heavy drinkers. Of women who drink, 63 percent are light drinkers and 37 percent are moderate or heavy drinkers. When you get into the heavy-drinking category, you find that this country has an estimated 9 million alcoholics.

Those nine million people are in a difficult situation—but fortunately, the medical community has recognized the fact that alcoholism is a disease, and diseases can be both cured and prevented. As we well know by now, prevention is by far the better way.

Many people throughout history have believed that the best prevention in this case is total abstinence, never to drink alcohol at all. But alcohol also has built-in health benefits as well as a long history of use as medicine. There are many cases in which moderate amounts of alcohol are good for you, and it can play an important role in the prevention of degenerative diseases.

How can it do this? An editorial in the doctors' newspaper *Medical Tribune* pointed out that "A ccuple of ounces of alcohol daily may be associated beneficially with higher level of HDL cholesterol—the good cholesterol that seemingly is protective against myocardial infarction." That's not one person's opinion but a finding based on years of scientific research. But please note that they said "a couple of ounces daily." That does not mean a three-martini lunch, a six-pack of beer at the ball game or half a magnum of champagne shared during a romantic interlude. It means two ounces, period.

The editorial went on to emphasize another well-known fact: "Alcohol is not a food. . . . It is a drug . . . described as 'the most abused drug in the United States.' " As a result of overuse of alcohol, "more than half of all highway accidents are alcohol-related; about half of the pedestrians killed in city streets are intoxicated; over 50 percent of crimes are associated with the use of alcohol." And far too many of us have personal experience with the disasters that overindulgence in alcohol can wreak on families and personal relationships.

I don't mean to scare you with all these grim facts. I do mean to make a strong point about the importance of moderation. It's a point I had to stress heavily with a patient of mine who was missing out on the good news because the bad news scared him nearly to death.

Mr. J. was a very successful advertising executive who had paid for his success with his health. Advertising is an extremely tension-filled business, and the tension was taking its toll on his heart. Every time he ate, he suffered severe attacks of angina pectoris—chest pain that results from poor circulation in the coronary arteries. After a while he became afraid to eat, knowing that every meal would be followed by pain that literally doubled him over. He ate so little that he lost more than 30 pounds and was badly underweight (not to mention weak and exhausted) when I saw him.

After I had examined Mr. J. and determined the nature of his problem, I urged him to drink one ounce of brandy or whiskey before his lunch and dinner, or to have two glasses of wine with the meal. I knew the alcohol would act as a tranquilizer. But my advice went over like the proverbial lead balloon.

It turned out that Mr. J.'s father had been an alcoholic, and that had resulted in his having been brought up in a broken home. Like many children of alcoholics, he had overreacted and vowed never to touch alcohol; he seemed to think that if he took so much as one drink he, too, would become an alcoholic.

After a lot of explaining and persuading, I finally convinced Mr. J. to take my advice and think of his drinks as medicine prescribed by his physician. There was, of course, a small risk involved—some people in these circumstances will find that they like liquor so much that they *do* become alcoholics. But I didn't think Mr. J. was the type to do that, and I was right. He did not become an alcoholic. He drank only the amount I had advised, and the treatment worked beautifully. After several months he was back to his normal weight, and a wonderful change had taken place in his personality. He was much less tense (and therefore much more efficient in his work, which contributed to a further decline in tension), he took life a little less seriously, he began to appreciate himself more and he was able to eat normal, healthy meals with only an occasional twinge of what had formerly been truly awful pain. The moderate amount of alcohol had eased the tension that was interfering with his digestion and placing a severe strain on his heart.

The moral of the story is that a moderate amount of alcohol is a blessing, but a large amount is a curse. Nature has its own way of bringing this fact home, even before you reach the danger point: If you drink a moderate amount of alcohol, you feel fine; if you drink too much, you get a hangover.

Let's look at some specifics.

What Can Alcohol Do for You?

It can relax you. As in the case of Mr. J., alcohol can act as a very helpful relaxant. This surprises a lot of people, since their own experience tells them that they feel energetic and jolly or "pepped up" after a couple of drinks. But you have to be emotionally relaxed before you can feel jolly and pepped up—and much of your reaction to alcohol depends on the circumstances in which you drink it. If you're at a party or having a few drinks in a pub with good friends, the mood is cheerful, and the relaxing effect of alcohol helps you to forget your problems and slip into that cheerful mood. On the other hand, we've all heard about the miserable soul who's just been fired or lost his best friend and goes into a dark, dreary bar to sit alone and drown his sorrow. His psychological state is so poor that the drinks relax him into more self-pity; pretty soon he's crying into his beer (or worse, something stronger) and pouring out his tale of woe to a bored bartender. If he gets drunk enough, the alcohol will wash all his troubles away, relaxing him so much that he'll pass out. But when he wakes up, the troubles will be as bad as ever, compounded by his hangover.

Alcohol, then, is not a stimulant but a depressant. It does relax you, but again the key is moderation. A little relaxation is good for you, but this, too, can be overdone.

It can help your digestion. Why has it become a custom for people to have a drink or two before dinner? Because the alcohol relaxes not only your mind, but your stomach muscles, making your digestion far more efficient. It also stimulates your appetite, which is like priming the pump for the meal. This, of course, has to be taken into consideration by people who need to lose weight, and they also have to be very aware of the high amounts of calories in alcoholic beverages, as we'll see later. But unless you're on a weight-loss diet, the pre-dinner drink should stimulate you to eat the right amounts of the foods you know are good for you.

Moderate amounts of alcohol also stimulate your kidneys, which is very important to good health.

It can help your circulation. Alcohol has long been known to doctors as a vasodilating agent—that is, a chemical that widens the veins and arteries and increases the flow of blood. Vasodilation is very important for people whose arteries have already been narrowed by arteriosclerotic plaques, but they represent severe cases, and a couple of drinks a day will not help them. For those people, doctors prescribe specific drugs that have a much stronger vasodilating effect.

For most people, however, alcohol in moderation acts as a gentle stimulant to the circulation that is very helpful. But too much brings about *over*stimulation: The blood vessels become overdilated, and when this happens to the vessels in the head, a person loses his judgment and coordination, gets dizzy and staggers, a condition on which society has put the fitting label, "drunk." The next day, the blood vessels become constricted as a reaction to having been overdilated, and that brings about the headache that is part of a hangover.

It can raise your HDL level. There was a time when scientists believed that alcohol acted as a solvent that would dissolve the saturated fat and arteriosclerotic plaques that block the arteries. It can, but only in enormous amounts, far too much for any human being to tolerate. That much alcohol would "pickle" your insides, and before it dissolved the dangerous cholesterol it would dissolve your liver first. However, you get a much better effect from the right amounts of alcohol.

We now know that alcohol in moderation can gently but surely increase the amount of the good cholesterol, HDL. This is the primary reason why, in terms of the Institute Program, a couple of glasses of wine with dinner are excellent for anyone who is able to stop at a couple and who is not on a weight-loss diet or subject to other restrictions.

The most important of these other restrictions is the diabetic diet. If you are diabetic, you already know that alcohol is very heavy in sugar content and must be carefully restricted or eliminated altogether. Some diabetics can drink a little alcohol, while others can't touch it at all. That's an individual matter that has to be determined by the diabetic's doctor. If you're playing host or hostess to a diabetic, don't urge him or her to have a couple of drinks because of what I've said about alcohol's benefits. A diabetic has to follow doctor's orders to the letter.

It can ease pain. While alcohol is relaxing your emotions and your stomach muscles, it's also relaxing your awareness of pain. In this respect it has a definite narcotic or analgesic effect.

This can be helpful to heart patients, but only to a degree, and again there is an element of risk. For a long time it was thought that the pain of angina was relieved by alcohol because of the solvent or vasodilating effects already described. But these are not strong enough to eliminate the pain itself. What alcohol does is eliminate the patient's *perception* of pain and raise his pain threshhold.

Heart patients have to be warned about these effects and must take the warning seriously. It is of course desirable to lessen or eliminate pain. But pain is one of nature's most important warning signals—many heart patients have overexerted themselves and strained their hearts while under the influence of alcohol because the lack of pain, plus the general feeling of relaxation, made them think everything was all right. A heart condition is nothing to take chances with. If your doctor tells you that moderate alcohol and exercise are both good for you, that does not mean you should belt down a couple of Scotches, then jump out on the dance floor. Common sense is always important, but even more so when your body is already endangered.

On the whole, I find that alcohol in moderate amounts is an excellent relaxing agent for people with heart problems, as well as a mild vasodilator and a means of improving the ratio of HDL to LDL and VLDL cholesterol.

How Can Alcohol Harm You?

There's no need to expound on the evils and dangers of drunkenness, because everybody knows them. But here's an example of just how serious the consequences can be when drinking gets out of hand:

Legend has it that, on Christmas night, 1776, when George Washington made his historic crossing of the Delaware with a small band of battered, frozen and ill-fed men, the British were defeated because "Cornwallis' men had drunk not wisely, but too well." These words have been credited to the Father of Our Country himself. Can you imagine what might have happened if the enemy had been sober and alert? We might still be stopping for high tea and crumpets every afternoon and saluting the Union Jack.

How, specifically, can too much alcohol harm you?

It can "fry your brain." This slang expression simply means that an overload of alcohol can dull your senses, slow your reactions, reduce your ability to think clearly and even cause irreversible brain damage. As J. Cutting, M.D., put it so well in the *British Journal of Psychiatry* in 1978, "It is now recognized that heavy and prolonged alcohol intake can lead to a deterioration of mental functions."

As far back as 1883, the noted German pharmacologist Oswald Schmiedeberg wrote that an overdose of alcohol can result in "loud and profuse speech and vivacious acts, also to accelerated pulse rate, engorgement and flushing of the body surface and the face, and a sensation of increased warmth. . . . a closer consideration of these manifestations shows that they are the results of a beginning paralysis of certain parts of the brain."

Paralysis of certain parts of the brain! That's what the slang phrase "fry your brain" means. It takes quite a while and quite a lot of alcohol to bring things to that sorry a state, but anyone who cannot control the amount he drinks is well on the way to a degree of damage that can't be repaired.

It can hurt your circulation. This effect is just the opposite of what happens when you regulate your intake of alcohol; too much alcohol reverses the good that is done by a moderate amount through a process that some doctors have named a "coronary steal."

It was reported in the *American Journal of Cardiology* that for people who suffer from ischemic heart disease (in which some coronary arteries are too narrowed to permit a normal flow of blood), an excess of alcohol will increase the flow in the normal arteries by "stealing" blood away from the narrowed (ischemic) arteries. This creates a dangerous imbalance in the circulation.

It can contribute to malnutrition. Since I've already told you that before-dinner drinks can stimulate the appetite, you may wonder how alcohol can interfere with nutrition. The important factor is the amount of alcohol consumed. A lot of alcohol makes the drinker forget all about eating, so he skips his meal and goes right on drinking. When he wakes up with a hangover (part of which is an upset stomach), he has no desire for food, so he skips another meal and swallows only aspirin, antacids or a "cure" such as a Bloody Mary—which can start the drinking pattern all over again. If this happens often enough, the drinker will soon be malnourished.

Charles E. Becker, M.D., of San Francisco General Hospital, has put it very clearly: "Malnutrition is common among alcoholics because alcohol, which does not contain a significant amount of nutrients, displaces foods containing proteins, vitamins, and minerals. Chronic alcohol consumption also results in maldigestion and malabsorption of nutrients."

It can add excess weight. Alcohol contains no nutrition to speak of, but it does contain a lot of calories. What's worse, they are "empty" calories, the kind that are burned up or oxidized in the form of heat and cannot be converted into useful, healthy body tissue. You can gain weight by drinking a lot, but it will be useless, ugly fat.

Here's a list of most of the common alcoholic beverages and the approximate number of empty calories they contain:

ALCOHOLIC BEVERAGE	CALORIES
1 Tom Collins	180
1 3½-ounce highball	165
1 manhattan	164
3½ ounces of muscatel or port	158
1 martini	140
1 whiskey sour	138
1½ ounces of gin	104–133
1½ ounces of rum	104–133
1½ ounces rye whiskey	104–133
1½ ounces of Scotch	104–133
1 daiquiri	122
3½ ounces of wine	85
4 ounces of champagne	84
6 ounces of beer	76

SOURCE: Adapted from *Food Values of Portions Commonly Used* by Jean A. T. Pennington, et al. (New York: Harper & Row, 1980).

It can destroy your liver. Probably everyone has heard of cirrhosis of the liver, and most people think it is a direct result of alcoholism. This is not always the case. There are different types of cirrhosis of the liver, which is basically the outgrowth of a nutritional disorder. Therefore, when you hear that someone has cirrhosis of the liver, you should not automatically think that he's an alcoholic.

Nevertheless, it's a pretty good bet he is. *Most* cirrhosis of the liver is what doctors call alcoholic cirrhosis, but no one is really sure whether it is a direct result of alcohol's effect on the liver or is caused by the nutritional deficiency that so often accompanies chronic drinking. At this point, experiments with laboratory rats lean in favor of the nutritional deficiency being at fault.

In the early stages of the disease, the liver becomes enlarged and is engorged with fatty deposits. Later, the liver shrinks and becomes hard, which is characteristic of dying tissue. The liver is literally dying, and the body it occupies will also die if the disease is not stopped in time. The symptoms of cirrhosis range progressively from nervousness to fatigue to indigestion to vomiting and passage of blood to chest pain to abdominal pain and swelling to jaundice to coma and, finally, to death.

It takes a long time—years—for all this to happen. The disease can be cured if it is caught in time—and if the patient is able to stop drinking alcohol and improve his nutritional state. Some years ago I introduced a treatment for cirrhosis that was based on a high-protein diet with the addition of nutritional and vitamin supplements as well as injections of liver extract (in line with my long-held theory of replacement therapy) and vitamins. I tested it with more than 100 patients and reported in the medical journals that it was temporarily effective as long as the patient stayed away from alcohol and maintained good nutrition. The treatment has been used extensively by doctors here and in other countries.

But the success of the treatment depends on the patient's cooperation. A person who drinks enough alcohol long enough to get cirrhosis of the liver is without question a chronic alcoholic, and that is a disease that is very difficult to cure. Success depends entirely upon the patient's desire to be cured, and there are no pills or injections that will give him a strong enough desire. I have found that even psychiatric treatment is useless in many cases.

Probably the best hope for an alcoholic (once he has made up his mind that he really wants to stay sober) is Alcoholics Anonymous, which has a very good record of helping people with this disease. This organization has been a blessing to countless unfortunate victims.

Needless to say, my advice about having a couple of glasses of wine with a meal does not apply to alcoholics—it's too easy to believe that, if a few drinks are beneficial, a few more can do no harm. The alcoholic who thinks this way will soon be off the wagon and back in trouble again. The use of alcohol has to be very carefully regulated by each individual; if you can't regulate it easily, *don't touch it!*

It can give you the DTs. "DTs" is a nickname for *delirium tremens,* a condition that often afflicts people who have been drinking heavily for a long time and suddenly try to stop. When the body has become accustomed to alcohol (as it will to any drug, no matter how dangerous) the patient who tries to "cold turkey" (quit suddenly) will go through very serious withdrawal symptoms. One of these symptoms is chilliness combined with bumpy skin resembling the skin of a plucked, uncooked turkey—that's where the term "cold turkey" comes from.

Another, and far more serious, symptom of withdrawal is delirium tremens, which is characterized by confusion, anxiety, feelings of persecution, hallucinations and delusions.

The DTs are an example of what can happen as a result of extreme overindulgence in alcohol. This condition will not affect anyone who drinks moderately, nor even the person who occasionally drinks too much and wakes up with a hangover. But it is a terrifying example of alcohol abuse.

Just how much is the difference between moderate use and abuse? And how much alcohol constitutes "moderate" drinking?

There is no definite answer because the tolerance to this substance varies so widely from person to person. Some people get giddy on a glass of wine or two; others seem to have the proverbial "hollow leg" and can put away enormous amounts without feeling or showing the effects. It can also depend on whether or not you are used to alcohol. Most people seem to have a fairly low tolerance when they are young and first experimenting with the "grown-up" practice of drinking. If they become accustomed to it, their tolerance increases, but only up to a point. When a person begins to abuse alcohol, his tolerance gradually decreases, until soon it takes only a drink or two to make him drunk.

A fatal dose of alcohol can be anywhere from 1 pint to 1 quart of whiskey or 8 to 16 ounces of pure alcohol. People who have died from acute alcohol intoxication have usually had blood levels of between 0.3 and 0.5 percent alcohol—and that is only a fraction of 1 percent. When people are given tests for drunken driving, the intoxication level in most states is set at 0.1 percent—only one-tenth of 1 percent.

What is the answer for you? There are two: (1) Alcohol taken in moderation is a good relaxant, a gentle helper for your circulation and a booster to your level of helpful HDL cholesterol—in short, good prevention; (2) alcohol taken in excess is a very dangerous poison. These are the facts. The way you use them is up to you.

Caffeine

Caffeine is the substance in coffee and tea that gives you that little "boost." But lately it's gotten a bad name. And for good reason. Caffeine is a stimulant to the nervous system, and too much of it can contribute to the tension that we know is harmful to our health. Caffeine also contributes to insomnia and the production of acid in the stomach, which can mean heartburn in normal people and devastating pain in those who have peptic ulcers. It has been linked to breast cancer in women and to birth defects in the children of women who drink too much coffee or tea during pregnancy.

All this sounds like yet another chamber of horrors, but please note that I said "too much." Once again we come back to the time-honored rule of moderation.

Coffee is without a doubt the most popular beverage in America. Most adults wouldn't think of starting the day without at least one cup, and many of them think they *couldn't*. They count on the stimulating effect of caffeine to wake them up, get them going, clear the cobwebs out of their heads, give them energy. That's the way a drug addict thinks about about his "morning fix."

In truth, most coffee drinkers are addicted to caffeine, either physically or psychologically, and both carry equal strength as forms of dependence. No healthy person should need a stimulant to get going in the morning. But we develop the coffee habit early in life, and soon we *believe* that we need it. That belief is as strong as any physical addiction.

Actually, the "energy" provided by caffeine is not real energy but nervous stimulation. Energy comes from calories, and coffee and tea have almost no calories until you put sugar and/or cream in the cup. Black coffee will stimulate you just as much as coffee laced with sugar and enriched with saturated-fat-filled cream.

This stimulation is not all bad, however. Mild caffeine stimulation is even helpful in some cases of heart disease, in circulatory disorders and in lung diseases. One of the derivatives of caffeine, called xanthine, is used in prescription drug form to treat these disorders. Nevertheless, a heavy coffee or tea habit can only do you harm.

By now you may be thinking, "Oh, no, just when I thought coffee was okay because it doesn't have any calories, I get hit with this!"

Relax. If you love the taste of coffee, there are now numerous decaffeinated brands that taste the same as real coffee. If you don't believe me, just watch television for a while. The knowledge of the dangers of caffeine has become so widespread that manufacturers have responded by decaffeinating their products and advertising them widely. If you still don't believe me, try one of the decaffeinated brands. If it tastes "funny" at first, that's because you know it's decaffeinated and you expect it to taste funny. Most of these brands are not fake coffee—they are real coffee with the caffeine removed. Caffeine has no taste, so the coffee flavor remains the same.

Still skeptical? Try it on someone you know is a coffee lover. Give him or her a cup of decaffeinated coffee without saying it's decaffeinated. Chances are the coffee lover won't know the difference!

"No matter how much it tastes the same," you're thinking, "it's not going to wake me up in the morning." You're right. You'll have to wake yourself up, and if you follow the Institute Program and get yourself in good shape, that won't be a problem; it will happen automatically. However, you may find it helpful to taper off your consumption of caffeinated coffee rather than trying to quit "cold turkey." And one or two cups of caffeine-containing coffee each day will not hurt you; they may even be beneficial as long as you stick to that "moderation" rule. If you love that coffee taste, and find the beverage helpful in getting you started (especially if you're one of those unfortunate people who "hate to get up in the morning"), I suggest that you buy both regular and decaffeinated coffee. Use the regular brand in the morning, then switch to the decaffeinated brand for the rest of the day. You can then have the best of both worlds!

Caffeine in Tea

A word about tea: This beverage is so popular in my native England that the English have an extra meal in the afternoon called "high tea." Everything stops around 3:30 or 4:00 P.M. while people relax with a cup of tea, often embellished with little sandwiches, pastries and scones. Obviously, this ritual is not good for the arteries, especially when butter-rich pastries are eaten. But the English are not going to give it up—it's a way of life. The compromise (and this goes for American tea lovers as well) is to drink decaffeinated tea and nibble on low-calorie, low-saturated-fat snacks.

The choice of decaffeinated teas is almost as wide as the choice of regular teas. My particular favorites are the herb teas—they come in a wonderful variety of flavors, have almost no calories or caffeine and are just as good iced as hot.

You may find the flavor of the herb teas so good that you won't even want a sweetener or cream substitute. Many people find that a slice of fresh lemon adds a refreshing taste to decaffeinated tea—and you get a little vitamin C as a bonus.

Like coffee, tea may be taken moderately in its caffeinated form—but I urge you to limit your intake to two or three cups a day, and drink decaffeinated tea the rest of the time.

Other Sources of Caffeine

If you read labels, you know that caffeine also exists in cola drinks. It may surprise you to learn that it is in cocoa and chocolate as well. Like coffee and tea, cola drinks are all right in moderation, though you should certainly stick to the low-calorie forms. And there are plenty of other delicious soft drinks and fruit juices that can satisfy your craving for a tall, cold, refreshing drink.

As for cocoa and chocolate, you know you shouldn't be eating much of these in candy and pastry form to begin with. In moderation they won't hurt. For a more healthful variety of chocolate, however, try mixing cocoa powder with polyunsaturated oil and a natural sweetener to make your own chocolate syrup without the butterfat and sugar that make the commercial brands so harmful. Add a little low-fat milk, and you have "milk chocolate!" Not bad for somebody who thought a healthy diet meant giving up all the good things in life.

On the cautionary side, as far as I know no one has yet put a decaffeinated cocoa on the market, so you do have to limit your consumption. But a cup of hot chocolate made with low-fat milk and a natural sweetener, a slice of homemade chocolate cake made with polyunsaturated fat and egg substitute or a spoonful of homemade chocolate syrup (made the way

I've described) over frozen vanilla yogurt are treats you will enjoy even more in moderation because you'll know how easily you're cheating degenerative diseases.

Tobacco

I promised I wouldn't tell you that you had to quit smoking in order to prevent a heart attack, and I won't. Plenty of people who've never smoked have had heart attacks, and some who've smoked all their lives have survived without a trace of either heart disease or lung cancer. As we all know, some folks are amazingly able to play with fire without getting burned.

But the odds are against you. Tobacco has now been implicated in a whole host of diseases including heart and blood-vessel disorders, cancer, emphysema, bronchitis, asthma and just recently, low birth weight in the infants of women who smoked during pregnancy.

The only good that smoking can do for you is psychological, not physical. (Physically, it is extremely damaging to your system.) Confirmed smokers will tell you firmly and stubbornly that cigarettes relax them—but it's not the cigarette that does the relaxing, it's the act of lighting and smoking it. The smoker sits back, takes out his cigarettes, puts one in his mouth, lights it, takes a deep drag, inhales and lets the smoke out with a relaxed and satisfied "ahhh." His tensions seem to float away with the smoke. But he could do the same thing with a breath of fresh air.

Smoking also gives people something to do with their hands. This is particularly helpful at social events, when one is meeting new people and may be nervous about not knowing what to do or say. So the nervous party-goer holds an alcoholic drink in one hand and a cigarette in the other and achieves a certain sense of calm. A nonalcoholic drink and a stick of celery would serve the same purpose.

Then there's the oral satisfaction of smoking. Many people just don't feel comfortable unless they have something in their mouths. That is why so many complain of gaining weight when they try to quit smoking. To satisfy their oral craving, they put anything into their mouths—and even chewing gum, unless it's sugar-free, is going to add excess calories if used as often as the smoker is accustomed to having his mouth occupied.

Finally, smoking may have become an addiction. If you're a smoker, you probably remember that when you first tried cigarettes you felt a little giddy and lightheaded when you lit up. That was the effect of nicotine, a drug that causes the blood vessels in your brain to dilate (expand) briefly. It gives you a momentary "high."

The brief high that you got from those first cigarettes disappeared pretty quickly, and soon it didn't happen at all, even when you lit up. Your system got so used to the nicotine that you didn't feel it anymore. But by that time, you probably noticed a desire for a cigarette after you hadn't had one for a while. The craving for a cigarette was part habit and part the beginnings of addiction.

Addiction? Absolutely. Nicotine is a drug, even though it is not a narcotic. Your body gets used to it, and when you stop supplying it for a while, your body wants more. It reacts the same way (though in a much stronger and more serious degree) to alcohol and even heroin. Your body needs you to do the thinking for it.

A longtime smoker who tries to quit abruptly will suffer withdrawal symptoms. Not as serious or as strong as the symptoms brought on by withdrawal from alcohol or narcotics, but sometimes pretty uncomfortable, they include nervousness, irritability, mouth watering, a bad taste in the mouth and the psychological feeling that something necessary is missing.

Some people can take the discomfort of withdrawal; others have a difficult time or find it impossible to tolerate. For those who have a hard time quitting the cigarette habit, numerous plans have been devised in the years since doctors realized how dangerous smoking is and the Surgeon General put that "harmful to your health" warning on all cigarette packs. These plans include the use of prescription or nonprescription medications that are supposed to ease the craving, sets of progressively stronger filters that allow you to get less and less of the nicotine, hypnotism, transcendental meditation, psychotherapy and group therapy in which hopeful quitters get together and apply the Alcoholics Anonymous principle of helping each other. Many of these are effective and have helped a lot of people give up the cigarette habit. But a small group of people just can't quit.

How to Cut Down on Cigarettes

I promised I wouldn't tell you that you had to quit smoking. But I will tell you that you absolutely should if you possibly can. If you really believe that you can't—if you are one of those people like Mark Twain, who said, "It's easy to quit smoking; I've done it hundreds of times!"—then you can do yourself and everyone around you a big favor by cutting down on the number of cigarettes you consume each day. Here are some ways you can make it easier:

Try not to inhale. This may be difficult at first, since you are probably used to pulling that smoke way down into your lungs before you blow it out. But try taking a shallow breath instead of a deep one whenever you are smoking. Try to keep the smoke in your mouth instead of "swallowing" it. The more you try it, the easier it will get. And you will still have the benefit of the tobacco taste you have grown to love.

Use a filtered cigarette holder. This serves a double purpose. First, it keeps a large amount of the nicotine and tar out of your system while allowing you enough to prevent withdrawal symptoms and loss of taste. Second, the plastic end of the holder acts as an "adult pacifier"—that is, it gives you something to hold in your mouth to satisfy that oral craving. You can hold the cigarette holder in your mouth as often or as long as you want, but how often you fill it with a cigarette should be a matter of careful thought.

Filtered cigarette holders come in a lot of varieties. Some are disposable and designed to be thrown away after a few cigarettes. Others are refillable—you buy the holder and the filters separately, and change the filter whenever you think you need a new one. If you want to see what cigarette smoking does to your lungs, keep a filter in the holder until you've finished a pack of cigarettes, then take it out and look at it. When you put it in, it was white. When you take it out, it's dark brown, crusted and sticky with all the tar and nicotine that would have gone into your body without the filter!

Best of all, in my opinion, are the progressive filters, designed to help you cut down your smoking to the point of quitting entirely. The first filter you put in the holder is relatively mild—you hardly notice the slight decrease in the amount of smoke you get. The next filter is a little bit stronger, the next one stronger yet, and so on until you gradually reach the point of inhaling very little smoke at all. By this time you're spending so much money on cigarettes and getting so little of what they "offer" that you might as well quit altogether. Your system will have tapered off so gradually that you won't feel any withdrawal effects. And nobody says you can't still keep the holder as a pacifier if you want to.

Be considerate of other people. If you're a smoker, you're probably sick and tired of all the complaining you've been hearing from nonsmokers and (worse!) ex-smokers. People who have given up a bad habit are certainly among the most holier-than-thou creatures in the world, and they just won't stop reminding you how much better off they are than when they were doing what you do. And have you noticed that "allergy" to smoke seems to have become a national epidemic? People who went along for years tolerating the smoking of others are now doubling over in exaggerated coughing spells, waving their arms in the air and protesting, "I'm allergic!" every time you light up.

That's because smoking has suffered a setback in social position. Whereas once it was considered a very adult, sophisticated and "cool" thing to do, now it is socially unacceptable. How often did you see Humphrey Bogart or Bette Davis without a cigarette? Not very often. But do modern stars smoke? Seldom if ever! Tough TV cops satisfy their oral cravings with lollipops, and high-fashion models make TV commercials to discourage teenagers from starting the smoking habit. Nowadays when you see someone smoking in movies or on TV, it's because it has something to do with the plot.

Now that smoking has a bad name, hordes of people are jumping on the bandwagon and boosting their own egos by claiming to be among the "good guys" who don't smoke. Actually, not many people are physically allergic to cigarette smoke. But if you don't smoke you know how *irritating* somebody else's smoke is, and the fact is that simply being near a smoker can be as harmful as smoking itself.

Cigarette smoke produces carbon monoxide, the same gas that comes out of the exhaust pipe of your car. If you want to commit suicide, you can close yourself in a car and run a hose from the exhaust pipe into the seating area. Enough carbon monoxide will kill you.

You cannot commit suicide by being around a smoker, but the amount of smoke that does get into your system does you no good. The smoke itself smells bad, can make you cough, and will make your eyes sting and water. Is it any wonder you don't want other people to smoke if you're not a smoker yourself?

If you're the smoker, have a heart—your own heart will benefit from it. Make a point of not smoking when you're around people who don't smoke. You can take it, and it will help you to cut down. When you're in a restaurant or a business meeting, you can always excuse yourself for a few moments if the urge becomes unbearable, but that will happen less and less and less often as you get used to abstaining. When you fly, try sitting in the no-smoking seats for a change; if the plane isn't full you can always change your seat later in order to prevent a "nicotine fit." Besides, the airlines make smokers sit in the back of the plane, where they must endure loud engine noise, get their meals last, and are delayed in getting off the plane when it lands.

How to Quit for Good

After you've tried one or all of these cutting-down methods for a while, you may find that you would like to quit altogether. Bravo! Your heart, your lungs and most likely your family will be much the better for it. And you will have taken a big step toward putting degenerative diseases into reverse gear.

One of the best plans for quitting smoking that I have come across was described in *Modern Medicine* (October, 1981) by two smoking specialists who say that it's important to *prepare* to quit as well as to avoid cravings.

To prepare yourself to stop smoking, they say, first set a quitting date. Then take the time to do a little paperwork: Make lists of why you smoke, why you *don't* quit and why you *should* quit. Write down what you think are the benefits of becoming a nonsmoker. List each and every cigarette you smoke for two weeks. And keep a running list of what triggers your smoking; anything that sets off the urge to smoke qualifies, such as a martini or a cup of coffee. If just the sight of an ashtray triggers the urge, add it to your list. Situations count, too. If you reach for a cigarette before meeting a client, whenever the phone rings or the second after eating the last bite of dinner, make a note of it.

Next, take a long, hard look at all those lists you drew up. They're for you—because part of the battle lies in clarifying your own motives and in identifying exactly what makes you vulnerable. Once you pinpoint the behavior patterns linked to being a smoker, you can work at breaking them to become a nonsmoker. It's like having a map to tell you where the quicksand lies so that you can get around it.

Although you can't avoid the situations that trigger your smoking, such as talking on the telephone or meeting a client, you *can* stock up on oral satisfiers as substitutes for smoking. Try sunflower seeds, toothpicks or sugarless gum—whatever works. Also, let activities such as walking or tennis be a release for your energy. Be sure to tell your friends you're quitting, and ask for their help. (Maybe you'll find a new racquetball partner or two!)

One device that you should make for yourself is a smoking jar. The smoking experts ask first that you place two weeks' worth of cigarette butts in this jar. When you quit, flood the butts with water and cover the jar; whenever you get a craving for a smoke, sniff the awful aroma of the butts in the jar.

Once you have stopped smoking, fight those inevitable cravings with psychological warfare. Concentrate away your cravings with these recommended slogans:

- One smoke, one smoker.
- I have the strength to do it.
- A craving for a cigarette will go away whether or not I smoke a cigarette.

Or look around you and name objects as a distraction technique. The researchers say that a craving should subside by the time you've found twelve objects, using the phrase, "Now I'm aware of _____." You can also daydream away those urges, first by imagining a negative scene connected with smoking (fifteen seconds, eyes closed), then by imagining a pleasant scene as a self-reward.

The experts also advise you to shout out "Stop!"—when you "need" a cigarette. Such a technique is great if you're in your car out on the freeway, but if you're at the movies, no one's going to be sympathetic with your quitting campaign. Learn to shout silently, or try taking a deep breath through your mouth, hold it for a few seconds and then exhale slowly.

After a year is up, you award yourself a cash prize—because all through your efforts to stop smoking you have put in your piggy bank what you would have put into the tobacco manufacturer's pocket. Use that money for something you *really* want. You deserve it.

Smokers that have kicked the habit have good reason to feel as though they've given themselves a "new lease on life." Smoking, as you are aware, is one of the controllable risk factors in heart disease. Known for a long time to be true for men, a study by Walter C. Willett, M.D., of Harvard Medical School has shown that this fact is just as true for women. But Dr. Willett's study also showed that people who *quit* smoking (unless they already have irreversible emphysema or lung cancer) do not retain the bad effects of this harmful habit.

Dr. Willett found that the risk of myocardial infarction (heart attack) among smokers was three times greater than the same risk among nonsmokers. If they smoked two or more packs a day, the risk was *five* times greater. But the risk among people who had quit smoking was *no greater* than the risk among nonsmokers.

This benefit is the same as the benefit you can give your heart and arteries by changing from a high-saturated-fat diet to a low-saturated-fat diet and taking the Institute Formula *before* you get arteriosclerosis. There is a point of no return. Turn back before you reach it, and you should never have to face the degenerative diseases that wait at the end of the road.

Millions of persons in the United States in 1981 showed that they could stop smoking at a certain time and date and even refrain from smoking entirely. The American Cancer Society reported on its "smoke-out" in the *Los Angeles Times* of November 18, 1982 as follows:

> *One million smokers in California—including virtually the entire population of the town of Solvang— were expected to stop puffing at least today as part of the American Cancer Society's Seventh Annual 'Great American Smokeout.' The society said that last year an estimated 4.5 million Americans stopped smoking for the 24-hour period, and a Gallup Poll showed that 2.7 million still were not smoking 10 days after the event.*

The Triple Play

Alcohol, caffeine and tobacco, when used in excess, present a definite, documented triple threat to your health. Used in moderation, alcohol and caffeine can be beneficial to health, while tobacco can be reduced from a potent to a mild threat. It's up to you.

In baseball, when you get three runners out at the same time, it's called a triple play and is a cause for heavy celebration by the team that can pull it off. If you can pull off your own triple play against alcohol, caffeine and tobacco, you've got the stuff winners are made of!

Chapter 9

THE INSTITUTE PROGRAM— A PEACEFUL WEAPON

Having read almost all of this book, you now have in your head as well as in your hands one of the most powerful defensive weapons man has ever devised. It is unique in that category because, while most weapons are based on the principle of injury or death of an enemy, this weapon is based on preservation of *life*—yours. Because it is designed not to repel an attack but to prevent that attack in the first place, the Institute Program can truly be called a *peaceful weapon*.

The enemy, of course, is degenerative disease, a collective term that covers everything from obesity to malnutrition, poor circulation to arteriosclerosis. The battle is begun at birth (though it can be assumed at any time in life), the duration is as long as you live and the victory is long-lasting good health—measured graphically in the number of candles on your birthday cake each year and your ability to keep blowing them out even after there are enough to be considered a fire hazard!

I certainly don't expect you to remember all the details you've read in the previous chapters. They are there as evidence that all facets of the Institute Program have been scientifically tested and proven to be effective, and as reference material to which you can turn whenever you want to refresh your memory or prove a point to someone else. But I do expect you to remember the basic elements of this protective weapon. You don't have to know how to put a gun together in order to protect yourself with it, but you do have to remember where the trigger is and how to pull it.

Here, then, in review, are the basic points to remember in your peaceful war against premature aging and early death:

The Enemy	The Allies
Saturated fat	Polyunsaturated fat
LDL and VLDL	HDL
Stress	Relaxation through exercise
Lethargy	Activity
	The Institute Formula
	The Institute Diet

As you can see, the Institute Formula provides you with an extra (and very special) weapon that has never been available before. It's a bonus and a booster—and if you're old enough to have been under attack by the enemy for a long time (long enough to have lost a few battles), it can give you a brand-new fighting chance. Damage that has already been done *can* be repaired, up to a point. Unless you are already a victim of advanced arteriosclerosis, your chances of stopping the progress of degenerative disease are good.

But what if you're young, healthy, energetic and physically fit? Why should you bother with a special program of diet, exercise and the Institute Formula?

Because the enemy is just around the corner. The lifestyle modification that includes a low-saturated fat/calorie-regulated diet, individualized exercise and daily use of the Institute Formula sets up a barrier against hyperlipidemia and degenerative changes. And when you consider the fact that these disorders affect the majority of our population and are at least partially responsible for about 50 percent of the adult death rate in the United States and other Westernized countries, you know you are a born target.

About 50 percent—that's half the population! And look at the tie-in: As I pointed out in chapter 2, we know that about half our children, from ages 6 to 16, already have fatty streaks in their coronary arteries and aortas.

If they have inherited "good" genes—protective, healthy, defensive genes—from their parents and ancestors, these fatty streaks will be metabolized or burned up. Pathologists find that this happens in many cases because of healthy amounts of the protective cholesterols, HDL, phospholipids, LDL receptors and phosphatides, which are inherited through the "good" genes on the blueprint of the genetic code that determines all our characteristics.

The balance of the people, however, will go on to suffer and eventually die too early from the degenerative diseases that lead to arteriosclerosis, heart attack and stroke—*unless* they fight back.

Therefore, it is never too soon to begin building defenses. Start with number one—yourself. Once you've personally experienced an improvement in your own health and feelings of well-being, you'll be even better equipped to share the Institute Program with your family and other loved ones. You may have to "sell" it to them, but the best salesman is the person who believes in his product.

If you have children, you can control their diets at least to some extent. You may not be able to keep them away from junk food entirely, but you can see to it that they get the right amounts of the right foods as well—and most children don't have to be concerned with calories, since their natural activity and energy burn them up so quickly. In children, exercise usually takes care of itself. And you can see to it that your youngsters take the Institute Formula every day just as you do; you'll be giving them a head start in their defense against degenerative diseases, a head start that no generation before them has ever had.

In the adult world, I know from experience that there are two groups when it comes to preventive medicine: those who care and those who don't. The first group, those who care, are the ones who will see a doctor for a physical checkup, a weight analysis, calorie and exercise recommendations and blood tests that include a blood-lipid determination; they will ask for a breakdown of HDL, LDL and VLDL as well as a total cholesterol count. Then they will follow their doctor's advice and increase their chances for a longer and healthier life.

The second group (unfortunately, this group is larger than the first) will dismiss preventive medicine as being a lot of nonsense. They may even see it as a scheme by doctors to get healthy people to come for examinations they don't really need. But that idea doesn't make sense. The healthier you are, the *less* often you'll need to see a physician—and no doctor ever got rich on physical examinations and blood-lipid determinations alone. The second group spends a lot more on doctors and hospitals in their later years, when the lack of preventive medicine has left them vulnerable to the enemy and they have become the victims of debilitating and fatal diseases.

I'm happy to say that the first group is getting bigger all the time. People are more optimistic and less fatalistic than they used to be. They look at history and see that 100 years ago the average person's life expectancy was thirty-five to forty years, but now, in the 1980s, it's seventy to seventy-five years. And the past 100 years has been the time when medicine has made its greatest advances, the time when preventive medicine has come into its own and been recognized as a legitimate branch of science. People today realize that they are *not* powerless against degenerative disease, that they *can* have a voice in their own fates.

We doctors know we'll never be able to convince everyone. But the steady growth of the first group is more than just encouraging, it's cause for celebration. That means you have good cause to celebrate, too—you must be in the first group, or you wouldn't be reading this book. Here's to you!

Before I present you with a step-by-step plan for following the Institute Program, I'd like to include a few words about an element of good health that has so far been mentioned just in passing but deserves more attention: vitamins.

How to Use Vitamins

I haven't said much about vitamins because you get all (or most of) the vitamins you need from what you eat—if you follow a good, balanced, nutritious diet and don't boil the nutrition out of your food. But, in many cases, people who think they are in "good health" actually have a subclinical—or unnoticeable—vitamin deficiency that is slowly contributing to the development of a degenerative disease. Taking a multivitamin is a harmless way to minimize this risk.

Evidence that many diseases may be caused by inadequate diets has been available for centuries. As far back as 1753, a British naval surgeon named James Lind discovered that scurvy, a disease that afflicted seamen on long voyages and sometimes killed entire crews, could be cured by the eating of fresh limes or lemons. What's in limes and lemons (and other citrus fruits, as well as strawberries)? Vitamin C, although Dr. Lind didn't know that's what was curing the sailors.

A century later, a Japanese naval doctor learned that beriberi, a wasting disease that was striking down Japanese sailors right and left, could be eliminated by a change of diet. Other medical researchers began reporting similar results in using diet and dietary supplements to cure deficiency diseases, including rickets. But their discoveries were largely ignored. As late as the turn of the twentieth century, physicians of good educational background and wide experience were still blaming rickets on nonnutritional causes such as infection, lack of proper thyroid function and insufficient exercise. Why? That's a very good question that has never been answered. Maybe they just thought that diet was too simple a remedy and that anything so easy was too good to be true.

Finally, in 1906, the medical profession began to sit up and take notice of the effects vitamins and nutrition could have on health. At that time a British biochemist, Sir Frederick Gowland Hopkins, published the results of experiments that pointed clearly to the existence of vitamins. Sir Frederick had fed laboratory rats a diet of protein, fats and carbohydrates. He gave them plenty of food, so they should have grown satisfactorily. But instead, they became ill.

When he added milk to the rats' diets, however, they recovered quickly and began to grow normally. This result convinced Sir Frederick that a healthful diet needs not only adequate amounts of proteins and carbohydrates, but some unknown essential ingredients as well.

What were these ingredients? A Polish biochemist named Casimir Funk, who carried on similar research, gave them a name: vitamins.

But what were these "vitamins"? At first medical scientists thought they were bio-catalysts, which are substances that activate chemical reactions in the body without taking a direct part in these reactions. Today we know that vitamins often do more than just activate chemical reactions. Some of them may actually be substances that the body uses in forming its tissues and structures.

We certainly don't know everything about vitamins, even today. But we do know that there are (at least for now) over a dozen vitamins that are considered essential for a healthy body. Of these, the Institute Program is most concerned with the group of vitamins known as "B complex," and with vitamins A and C.

B complex vitamins supply us with a number of substances that are usually regarded as necessary for good health. They are vital to normal metabolism and are also very valuable as "lipotropic" or fat-fighting agents—good weapons in the battle against degenerative diseases that lead to arteriosclerosis, heart attack and stroke. In addition to helping our bodies fight saturated fats, certain of the B complex vitamins also act as "spark plugs" to our necessary hormones and help to prevent diseases of the nervous system.

B vitamins occur naturally in leafy green vegetables, which are also very low in calories and high in fiber. There you have three excellent reasons for eating lots of leafy green vegetables—and for *not* boiling the vitamin B out of them.

Vitamin A is essential for growth, for many bodily functions in the skin and blood vessels and for resistance against colds and other infections. It is a yellow compound related to substances found in carrots and leafy vegetables, so it's no surprise that you get a good supply of it by eating those foods—unboiled, of course.

Vitamin C is needed for formation of connective tissues and red blood cells. A deficiency may be partly responsible for, among other things, dental cavities and infections of the gums, for a loss of appetite and for anemia.

Vitamin C occurs naturally in citrus fruits (oranges, lemons, limes, tangerines, grapefruit) as in strawberries and broccoli. However, the vitamin is a crystalline substance that is very easily destroyed by cooking. In addition, the body cannot store vitamin C, so your supply needs to be renewed every day.

If you live where citrus fruits grow on trees, and you're particularly fond of them, you may get enough vitamin C if you eat these fruits raw or drink their fresh juices every day. But even Californians and Floridians may get tired of eating and drinking the same fruits and juices all the time. So I recommend that you take a good multivitamin tablet that includes vitamin C.

In addition to these vitamins, a number of minerals are also essential to a good diet, especially a diet aimed at preventing and fighting the degenerative diseases that lead to arteriosclerosis, heart attack, stroke and the premature aging that precedes them. You can get all these vitamins and minerals if you follow the dietary suggestions listed in chapter 5 of this book. But I know that you're human and that, like everybody else, you're going to want more variety in your diet—nobody uses just one cookbook, after all.

Therefore, my realistic advice is that you follow my dietary recommendations as much possible. Make sure you get enough protein, carbohydrate and good fats each day. Don't let yourself get careless about eating enough vegetables and fruits. Keep an eye on your calorie intake to be sure that you get enough calories, but not too many.

Then take a vitamin supplement. You may have heard that some vitamins can be dangerous if you take too large a dose, and that's true. But to take that much you would have to swallow whole handfuls of them. I'm suggesting that you take a reputable multivitamin tablet, one each day, in addition to (1) following the basic rules of my low-saturated-fat diet, and (2) taking the Institute Formula as directed. If you do that, you can't go wrong.

How to Follow the Institute Program

Now that you have all the background material, it's time to swing into action. You'll probably be surprised at how easy it is. And even after all I've told you, I'm sure you'll still be pleasantly surprised at the results.

Step 1. See your doctor for a complete physical checkup. After he or she has listened to your heart, taken your pulse and blood pressure, and examined your ears, nose and mouth, request blood-lipid profile tests. Explain why—and be sure to let your physician know that you want information and advice on the blood-lipid *fractions:* HDL, LDL and VLDL. He or she will probably be surprised to encounter such an informed patient.

Have your weight checked, and ask the doctor what your daily calorie intake should be, based on your height, weight, age, sex, bone structure and activity level. If you are normally an inactive person, mention that you plan to begin a program of regular exercise so that your calorie intake can be adjusted accordingly.

Ask for advice about exercise. The doctor will know about any health problems you may have that might limit the amount or type of exercise you should engage in. If you are more than 35 years old, you will be tested to see how your breathing and heart rates react to exertion. (If you are not tested, ask to be.) Work out with the doctor an exercise program that will be beneficial without aggravating any problems you may have, and one that will be pleasing to you as a regular activity without becoming a bore or an unwelcome obligation.

(**Important:** If you are a woman of childbearing age, do not delay seeing your doctor whenever you think you might be pregnant. Your diet and exercise will have to be adjusted to benefit the extra life you're nourishing.

Armed with your blood-lipid levels, calorie requirements and exercise advice, work out a diet based on my recommendations and an activity program based on the doctor's suggestions and your own preferences.)

Step 2. Take the Institute Formula daily as described in chapter 5.

Step 3. Add vitamin supplements to your diet. Stay away from the cheap preparations that provide only small and practically useless quantities of vitamins and will have little effect on your health.

If you follow my dietary suggestions, you should take the following quantities of vitamin supplements each day:

Vitamin A	10,000 international units
Vitamin B_1	2.50 milligrams
Vitamin B_2	3.00 milligrams
Vitamin B_6	3.00 milligrams
Vitamin B_{12}	10.00 micrograms
Vitamin C	500 milligrams
Vitamin D	400 international units
Vitamin E	100 international units

Isn't that more than the minimum daily requirements recommended by the U.S. Food and Drug Administration? It sure is. But you're not the average person, remember? You're an individual, a health- and nutrition-conscious individual, and one who is waging an active defensive battle against degenerative diseases. These amounts will help to strengthen your defenses, and there is absolutely no way they can hurt you.

Step 4. Make sure you get 2 tablespoonsful of polyunsaturated fats each day. These can be taken in the form of salad dressings made with vegetable oil (preferably soybean oil), polyunsaturated margarine as a spread on bread or rolls, peanut butter or cooking oil. Remember that olive oil is neutral—2 tablespoonsful of it will not give you the amount of polyunsaturated fat you need. And even if you cook in oil, you will not get all the oil you use, since some will be left in the pan. The best way to get your daily requirement of polyunsaturated fat is in salad dressing or in margarine used as a substitute for butter. They are excellent replacements for the butter, cream, whole milk and egg yolks you have eliminated from your diet.

Step 5. Include in your diet 2 to 4 tablespoonsful of whole wheat germ each day. It may be eaten with cereal and fruit as a breakfast food, sprinkled on a salad or mixed in with the sauce or gravy you use in a main course. Wheat germ is very rich in both protein and vitamin B and is an invaluable addition to a healthful diet.

Step 6. Make sure your diet includes at least one 8-ounce glass of low-fat or nonfat milk each day, or use the equivalent amount on cereal, in cooking or in your coffee and tea. Milk has been called "the perfect food," but that's not quite correct. Nothing that contains as much saturated fat as whole milk does can be called perfect. But get rid of that saturated fat, and milk comes pretty close.

That's the Institute Program. It's not very detailed because the details are different for each individual, and you have to determine (with your doctor) which elements are the best for you and you alone. The basic program is very simple, like a house that has been built on a solid foundation but looks like every other house on the block. It's up to you to add the personal touches that will make it just right for you.

It's been said that you can never be too rich or too healthy. I know some people who are too rich for their own good, but do you think anyone could ever be too healthy? I don't. Try to be as healthy as you can possibly be!

Chapter 10

LONGER LIFE THROUGH MEDICAL PROGRESS

There you have it: the Institute Program, the story of the Institute Formula and my reasons for believing they can protect you from the degenerative diseases that lead to arteriosclerosis, heart attack and stroke.

As I stated in the beginning of this book, there are no guarantees in the field of health. I cannot and will not promise that you, as an individual, will never have a heart attack or will live to be 100—there are too many factors involved. But the Institute Program and Institute Formula can increase the *probability* that you'll live a long life, free of some of the most dangerous threats to your health and happiness.

How long can you live? No one knows for sure. But statistics show that human life expectancy has increased dramatically, and the largest increases have taken place in this century, the eighty-odd years in which all forms of science have gone from a slow but steady pace of progress to great leaps and bounds toward the future. For thousands of years man tried to figure out how to fly without success. Then, in a twentieth century spurt of progress, we not only invented the airplane but sent manned rocket ships to the moon. Medicine has followed this burst-of-progressive-energy trend, and a remarkable increase in longevity has been one of the results.

At the time of the Greek and Roman empires, the average life span was about thirty years. In this century we have coined the slogan "Life Begins at Forty"—in those days, most people didn't even live that long!

By the year 1900, the average life span was still less than fifty years. In approximately two thousand years, longevity had progressed only about twenty years. Today the average life span is about seventy-five years—a leap of twenty-five years in eighty years of one century.

There's no mystery about why or how this happened. The answer is medical progress, helped out by advances in sanitation and nutrition.

At the turn of the century, there was nothing unusual about a woman giving birth to twelve or more children during her childbearing years. But many of those children were born dead or died before their first birthdays, creating a very high infant mortality rate. Women of those days *expected* to go through twelve or more pregnancies in order to have four or five living offspring. Then medical techniques improved so dramatically that by 1960 we were marketing birth-control pills to try to curtail a population explosion. Today most families have two or three children, the majority of whom live to become adults.

There are many more examples. Before the turn of the century most surgeons were still operating while wearing their street clothes and without having washed their hands. That was because they didn't know about germs—and a great many surgical patients survived their operations only to die of infections. Smallpox, typhoid, tuberculosis, scarlet fever, tetanus and diphtheria killed thousands of people then; so did influenza (the flu), which created a deadly epidemic as recently as 1969. Remember the polio scare of the 50s, when children were warned to stay away from public swimming pools because their parents feared they'd get the crippling and sometimes fatal disease? Today we have vaccines against all these afflictions, and even against measles!

This history is presented just to show you how great medical progress has been during the twentieth century. I believe that the Institute Program and its star, the Institute Formula, are additional pages in that book of progress.

But my belief isn't based on fond hopes or wild guessing. It's based on facts, the results of the Institute's many experiments with heart patients. I recently asked one of the Institute's statisticians—Norbert H. Enrick, Ph.D., a professor at Kent State University and a world authority in his field—to analyze the results of four of these studies: on patients who took choline, on patients who followed a low-fat diet, on patients who

PROBABLE LIFE-EXTENSION FOR THOSE WHO FOLLOW THE INSTITUTE PROGRAM

THOSE IN GOOD HEALTH			THOSE WITH HEART DISEASE		
	Increased Longevity			Increased Longevity	
Age	Men	Women	Age	Men	Women
45	7.2 years	8.5 years	45	10.8 years	12.7 years
50	7.1	6.8	50	10.6	10.2
55	9.0	5.3	55	13.5	7.9
60	8.3	4.0	60	12.5	6.0
65	7.5	3.8	65	11.2	5.7
70	6.8	3.6	70	10.2	5.4
75	6.0	3.4	75	9.0	5.1

NOTE: Prepared by Norbert H. Enrick, Ph.D., Professor of Statistics at the Business School of Administration at Kent State University, Ohio, 1981.

took mucopolysaccharides (MPS) and on patients who took the Institute Formula. (See the four studies in Appendix.) Here is what he found: There is a possibility that by following the Institute Program both healthy people and heart patients will add extra years to their life—will, in short, increase their life expectancy. The preceding chart gives you an idea of how many extra years I'm talking about; as you see, it's quite a remarkable number. A fifty-five-year-old man with heart disease, for example, oculd expect ot live 13.5 extra years. (Bear in mind that this is an *average*.) Let me give you two actual examples of people who have followed the Institute Program with impressive results.

Dr. K. is a professor in a world-renowned university. At the age of 49, he had already experienced several strokes, a heart attack and other complications of circulatory disease. Obviously, it was virtually impossible for him to teach any longer, and his case had been pronounced hopeless by two of the most famous clinics in the world.

By good fortune, a physician he knew suggested that he visit our Institute, and he began to follow the Institute Program.

As I write this, Dr. K. has been free of his cardiovascular symptoms for thirteen years. He was awarded a prize as the university's best teacher; for exercise, he swims in the ocean, hikes in the countryside and recently has taken to mountain climbing—all at 62 years of age.

Another scientist I know had a serious heart seizure in 1949. According to statistics for his age and condition, he had six more years to live. But by religiously following the Institute Program, he is now more active than ever in his research career—*and he has had a gain in life and health of an astonishing and unprecedented twenty-eight years.*

You could do the same for your health. Notice I use the word "could." Neither I nor anyone else can guarantee that you'll definitely add healthful years to your life if you follow the Institute Program. But the scientific facts say that you can. And I certainly hope that you can. I wish you all success!

Appendix

FOUR STUDIES

COMPARISON OF SURVIVAL RATES OF PATIENTS WITH CORONARY THROMBOSIS WITH AND WITHOUT CHOLINE TREATMENT AFTER THREE YEARS

Deaths in 115 Choline-Treated Patients	Deaths in 115 Non-Choline-Treated Patients
14	35

SOURCE: Study conducted at the Los Angeles County General Hospital and Loma Linda University School of Medicine by William F. Gonzalez, M.D. and Lester Morrison, M.D., 1946–1949. Results originally published in the *American Heart Journal*, July/August, 1949, p. 729.

COMPARISON OF SURVIVAL RATES IN PATIENTS WITH CORONARY THROMBOSIS AND INFARCTION ON THE INSTITUTE LOW-FAT DIET

	AFTER 3 YEARS			AFTER 8 YEARS			AFTER 12 YEARS		
	Deaths	Sur-vivors	%	Deaths	Sur-vivors	%	Deaths	Sur-vivors	%
50 patients on normal diet	15	35	70	38	12	24	50	..	..
50 patients on low-fat, low-choles-terol diet	7	43	86	22	28	56	31	19	38

SOURCE: Study conducted at the Crenshaw Hospital and the Loma Linda University School of Medicine, with Lester Morrison, M.D. as principal investigator, 1948–1960. Results originally published in the *Journal of the American Medical Association*, June 25, 1960.

ACUTE CARDIAC INCIDENTS OCCURRING IN 60 MUCOPOLYSACCHARIDES-TREATED PATIENTS AND 60 CONTROL PATIENTS DURING A SIX-YEAR STUDY PERIOD

	MYOCARDIAL INFARCTIONS		Acute Coronary Insufficiency	Myocardial Ischemia	Total
	Fatal	Nonfatal			
Male:					
MPS	2	0	1	0	3
Controls	8	6	6	0	20
Female:					
MPS	2	0	1	0	3
Controls	6	4	6	6	22
All:	4	0	2	0	6
Controls	14	10	12	6	42

SOURCE: Study conducted at the University of California Center for Health Sciences, Kent State University, and the Institute for Arteriosclerosis Research by Norbert Enrick, M.D. and Lester Morrison, M.D., 1967–1973. Results originally published in *Angiology*, May, 1973, p. 269.

EFFECTS OF INSTITUTE NUTRITIONAL SUPPLEMENT ON PATIENTS WITH CORONARY HEART DISEASE (MORRISON GOLDMAN SERIES—THREE YEAR STUDY)

Number of Patients	Average Age	SEX Male	Female	Average Duration of Illness	EFFECT OF TREATMENT Improved	Unchanged	Worsened
118	62	87	30	6 years	88	24	1*

SOURCE: Based on the results of a study entitled "Reduction of Coronary Heart Disease Mortality by Nutritional Supplements," conducted in Great Britain by Carl Goldman, M.D., in conjunction with Lester Morrison, M.D., in the United States, 1978–1981.
*One patient (age 81) died following strenuous physical exercise.

COMPARISON OF CHD DEATHS IN PATIENTS TAKING INSTITUTE NUTRIENTS VS. CHD CONTROL PATIENTS TREATED CONVENTIONALLY[a]

Period of Study	Number of Patients[b]	DEATHS INS Treated[c]	Controls	Ratio INS-Treated vs. Controls
3 years	118	1	15	1:15

SOURCE: Based on the results of a study entitled "Reduction of Coronary Heart Disease Mortality by Nutritional Supplements," conducted in the United States by Lester Morrison, M.D. in conjunction with Carl Goldman, M.D., in Great Britain, 1978–1981.
[a]CHD = coronary heart disease.
[b]118 patients: 65, United States; 53, England.
[c]INS = institute nutritional supplement. Amount INS taken daily at meals = 15–30 grams (one to two rounded tablespoonsful).

REFERENCES

Chapter 3

American Heart Association. *Heartbook.* New York: E. P. Dutton, 1980.

"The Best Medicine." *Time,* June 1, 1981, p. 59.

Crawford, Patricia B., et al. "Serum Cholesterol of 6-Year-Olds in Relation to Environmental Factors." *Journal of the American Dietetic Association,* January, 1981, pp. 41–46.

Enos, William F., et al. "Pathogenesis of Coronary Disease in American Soldiers Killed in Korea." *Journal of the American Medical Association,* July 16, 1955, pp. 912–14.

Johnson, Roger S. "Can You Alter Your Heart Disease Risk." *Journal of the American Medical Association,* May 15, 1981, pp. 1903–8.

Margolis, Simeon. "Managing Risk Factors to Reduce Coronary Artery Disease and Deaths." *Hospital Medicine,* April, 1981, pp. 26–37.

Strong, J. P., and McGill, H. C. "The Pediatric Aspects of Atherosclerosis." *Journal of Atherosclerosis Research,* vol. 9, 1969, pp. 251–65.

Williams, Roger R., et al. "Cancer Incidence by Levels of Cholesterol." *Journal of the American Medical Association,* January 16, 1981, pp. 247–52.

Chapter 4

Adlersberg, David, and Sobotka, Harry. "Effect of Prolonged Lecithin Feeding on Hypercholesterolemia." *Journal of Mt. Sinai Hospital*, vol. 9, 1943, pp. 955–56.

"At Sea for FMC," *Progress*, 1978.

Bartus, Raymond T. "Effects of Pharmacological Treatments on Learning and Memory in Animal Models." Paper presented at the International Study Group on the Pharmacology of Memory Disorders Associated with Aging, Zurich, Switzerland, April 3–5, 1981.

Bowyer, D. E. "Reduction of Endocytosis in Arterial Smooth Muscle Cells by Poly-unsaturated Lecithin." *Medizinische Welt*, vol. 30, 1979, pp. 1447–48.

Brattsand, Ralph. "Actions of Vitamins A and E and Some Nicotinic Acid Derivatives on Plasma Lipids and on Lipid Infiltration of Aorta in Cholesterol-Fed Rabbits." *Atherosclerosis*, July/August, 1975, pp. 47–61.

Bricklin, Mark. "Nature's Cholesterol Cops." *Prevention*, November, 1976, pp. 33–44.

Carlisle, Edith M. "Silicon as an Essential Element." *Federation Proceedings*, June, 1974, pp. 1758–66.

Dorland's Illustrated Medical Dictionary. 26th ed. Philadelphia: W. B. Saunders, 1981, p. 261.

Feltman, John. "Winning Hearts and Minds with Lecithin." *Prevention*, April, 1979, pp. 153–61.

"Gains Reported in Heart Disease." *New York Times*, October 15, 1965, p. 1.

Gershfeld, Norman L. "Selective Phospholipid Adsorption and Atherosclerosis." *Science*, May, 1979, pp. 506–8.

Glomset, John A. "Role of High Density Lipoproteins and Lecithin: Cholesterol Acyltransferase in Lipid Transport." *Circulation*, October, 1979, p. 11-2.

Kritchevsky, David, et al. "Experimental Atherosclerosis in Rabbits Fed Cholesterol-Free Diets: Effect of Lecithin." *Pharmacological Research Communications*, September, 1979, pp. 643–47.

Krumdieck, Carlos, and Butterworth, C. E. "Ascorbate-Cholesterol-Lecithin Interactions: Factors of Potential Importance in the Pathogenesis of Atherosclerosis." *American Journal of Clinical Nutrition*, August, 1974, pp. 866–76.

Levy, Robert I. "Drug Therapy of Hyperlipoproteinemia." *Journal of the American Medical Association*, May 24, 1976, pp. 2334–36.

Mervis, Ronald F. "Dietary Choline Modulation of Pyramidal Cell Dendritic Spine Population in Aging Mouse Neocortex." Paper presented at the International Study Group on the Pharmacology of Memory Disorders Associated with Aging, Zurich, Switzerland, April 3–5, 1981.

Morris, J. N., et al. "Vigorous Exercise in Leisure-Time and the Incidence of Coronary Heart Disease." *Lancet*, February 17, 1973, pp. 333–39.

Morrison, Lester M. "Peptic Ulcer Disappearance after Feedings of Normal Human Gastric Juice." *American Journal of Digestive Diseases*, October, 1945, pp. 323–27.

―――. "New Methods of Therapy in Cirrhosis of the Liver." *Journal of the American Medical Association*, June 21, 1947, pp. 673–76.

―――. "Effect of Choline on the Prevention of Experimental Atherosclerosis." *Geriatrics*, July/August, 1949, pp. 236–38.

―――. "Serum Cholesterol Reduction with Lecithin." *Geriatrics*, January, 1958, pp. 12–19.

Morrison, Lester M., and Gonzalez, William F. "Results of Treatment of Coronary Arteriosclerosis with Choline." *American Heart Journal*, May, 1950, pp. 729–36.

Norum, Kaare R. "Some Present Concepts Concerning Diet and Prevention of Coronary Heart Disease." *Nutrition and Metabolism*, vol. 22, 1978, pp. 1–7.

"Oral Therapy for Infarction Shows Promise in Early Test." *Medical Tribune*, June 12, 1974, p. 3.

Peeters, H., ed. *Phosphatidylcholine*. New York: Springer-Verlag, 1976.

Saba, Paolo, et al. "Effects of Soybean Polyunsaturated Phosphatidylcholine (LipoStabil) on Hyperlipoproteinemia." *Current Therapeutic Research*, August, 1978, pp. 299–306.

Schwarz, Klaus. "Silicon, Fibre and Atherosclerosis." *Lancet,* February 26, 1977, pp. 454–57.

Schwarz, Klaus, et al. "Inverse Relation of Silicon in Drinking Water and Atherosclerosis in Finland." *Lancet,* March 5, 1977, pp. 538–39.

Shekelle, Richard B., et al. "Diet, Serum Cholesterol and Death from Coronary Heart Disease." *New England Journal of Medicine,* January 8, 1981, pp. 65–70.

Sherman, Carl. "Silicon: Crucial for a Healthy Heart?" *Prevention,* August, 1978, pp. 90–94.

"Shortcut to Cutting Down Cholesterol." *Medical World News,* November 22, 1974, p. 38E.

Simons, L. A., et al. "Treatment of Hypercholesterolaemia with Oral Lecithin." *Australian and New Zealand Journal of Medicine,* June, 1977, pp. 262–66.

Stancioff, Dimitri J., and Renn, Donald W. "Physiological Effects of Carrageenan." In *Physiological Effects of Food Carbohydrates,* edited by Allene Jeanes and John Hodge. Washington, D.C.: American Chemical Society, 1975, pp. 282–95.

ter Welle, H. F., et al. "The Effect of Soya Lecithin on Serum Lipid Values in Type II Hyperlipoproteinemia." *Acta Medica Scandinavica,* vol. 195, 1974, pp. 267–71.

Tompkins, Ronald K., and Parkin, Lillie G. "Effects of Long-Term Ingestion of Soya Phospholipids on Serum Lipids in Humans." *American Journal of Surgery,* September, 1980, pp. 360–64.

Tyroler, H. A. "Epidemiology of Plasma High-Density Lipoprotein Cholesterol Levels." *Circulation,* November, 1980, pp. IV-1–IV-3.

Voss, Tom. "The Heartening News about Lecithin." *Prevention,* February, 1981, pp. 87–91.

Wilson, A. C., et al. "Lecithin in Hyperlipidemia." *American Journal of Clinical Nutrition,* April, 1980, p. 916.

Chapter 5

"Chondroitin Reduces 'Coronary Incidents'." *Journal of the American Medical Association,* August 24, 1970, p. 1254.

Miller, Orville H. "Nutritional Aspects of Mucopolysaccharides." In *Applied Nutrition in Clinical Practice*, edited by Michael Walczak and Richard P. Huemer. New York: Intercontinental Medical Book Corp., 1973, pp. 69–76.

Morrison, Lester M. "Treatment of Coronary Arteriosclerotic Heart Disease with Chondroitin Sulfate A: Preliminary Report." *Journal of the American Geriatrics Society*, July, 1968, pp. 779–85.

————. "Response of Ischemic Heart Disease to Chondroitin Sulfate A." *Journal of the American Geriatrics Society*, October, 1969, pp. 913–23.

————. "Therapeutic Applications of Chondroitin-4-Sulfate. Appraisal of Biologic Properties." *Folia Angiologica*, September 10, 1977, pp. 225–33.

————. "Atherosclerosis: Is It Preventable or Reversible?" *Journal of the International Academy of Preventive Medicine*, Winter, 1977, pp. 9–21.

Morrison, Lester M., and Goldman, Carl H. "Prevention of Coronary Heart Disease and Cardiac Arrhythmia by Natural Food Supplements." Mimeographed. Loma Linda, Calif.: Institute for Arteriosclerosis Research.

Morrison, Lester M., et al. "Effects of Acid Mucopolysaccharides on Growth Rates and Constituent Lipids of Tissue Cultures." *Proceedings of the Society for Experimental Biology and Medicine*, October, 1963, pp. 362–66.

————. "Prevention of Atherosclerosis in Sub-Human Primates by Chondroitin Sulfate A." *Circulation Research*, August, 1966, pp. 358–63.

————. "Inhibition of Coronary Atherosclerosis in the X-Irradiated, Cholesterol-Fed Rat by Chondroitin Sulfate A." *Proceedings of the Society for Experimental Biology and Medicine*, December, 1966, pp. 904–11.

————. "Treatment of Atherosclerosis with Acid Mucopolysaccharides." *Experimental Medicine and Surgery*, vol. 25, 1967, pp. 61–71.

————. "Prolongation of Thrombus Formation Time in Rabbits Given Chondroitin Sulfate A." *Journal of Atherosclerosis Research*, March/April, 1968, pp. 319–27.

————. "Prolongation of the Plasma Thrombus Formation Time of Dogs Administered Chondroitin Sulfates A and C." *Experimental Medicine and Surgery*, vol. 28, 1970, pp. 188–93.

———. "Prevention of Vascular Lesions by Chondroitin Sulfate A in the Coronary Artery and Aorta of Rats Induced by a Hypervitaminosis D, Cholesterol-Containing Diet." *Atherosclerosis,* July/August, 1972, pp. 105–18.

Murata, K. "Inhibitory Effects of Chondroitin Polysulfate on Lipemia and Atherosclerosis in Connection with Its Anticoagulant Activity." *Naturwissenschaften,* vol. 49, 1962, p. 1.

Ohdoi, S. "A Supplementary Study of Sulfated Mucopolysaccharides and Experimental Atherosclerosis." *Tokyo Journal of Medicine and Science,* vol. 67, 1959, p. 1291.

Oshima, Y., et al. "Clinical and Experimental Studies on Mucopolysaccharides (Mucopolysaccharides and Atherosclerosis)." In *Biochemistry and Medicine of Mucopolysaccharides,* edited by F. Egami and Y. Oshima. Tokyo: Maruzen, 1962, p. 259.

Osmundsen, John A. "Gains Reported in Heart Disease." *New York Times,* October 15, 1965, p. 1.

Schwarz, Klaus. "Silicon, Fibre and Atherosclerosis." *Lancet,* February 26, 1977, pp. 454–57.

Chapter 6

Levy, Robert I. "Drug Therapy of Hyperlipoproteinemia." *Journal of the American Medical Association,* May 24, 1976, pp. 2334–36.

Morrison, Lester M. "Arteriosclerosis: Recent Advances in the Dietary and Medicinal Treatment." *Journal of the American Medical Association,* April 21, 1951, pp. 1232–36.

Shekelle, Richard B., et al. "Diet, Serum Cholesterol and Death from Coronary Heart Disease." *New England Journal of Medicine,* January 8, 1981, pp. 65–70.

Chapter 8

"Alcoholism." *Medical Tribune,* September 23, 1981, p. 28.

Becker, Charles E. "Medical Consequences of Alcohol Abuse." *Postgraduate Medicine,* December, 1978, pp. 88–93.

Cutting, J. "Specific Psychological Deficits in Alcoholism." *British Journal of Psychiatry,* August, 1978, pp. 119–22.

Friedman, Howard S. "Acute Effects of Ethanol on Myocardial Blood Flow in the Nonischemic and Ischemic Heart." *American Journal of Cardiology*, January, 1981, pp. 61–62.

Roos, Leslie. "A Smoke-Ending Strategy That Works." *Modern Medicine*, October, 1981, pp. 69–70.

Willett, Walter C., et al. "Cigarette Smoking and Non-Fatal Myocardial Infarction in Women." *American Journal of Epidemiology*, May, 1981, pp. 575–82.

INDEX